Contents

Closing address

Promoting Sexual Health

Proceedings of the Second International Workshop on Prevention of Sexual Transmission of HIV and other Sexually Transmitted Diseases, Cambridge, 24-27 March 1991

...on For AIDS

...rity

COMMISSION
OF THE EUROPEAN
COMMUNITIES

...of Mrs Catherine Lalumière,
Secretary General of the Council of Europe

Promoting Sexual Health

Proceedings of the Second International Workshop on Prevention of Sexual Transmission of HIV and other Sexually Transmitted Diseases, Cambridge, 24-27 March 1991

A joint project of the British Medical Association Foundation for AIDS and the Health Education Authority

Edited by Hilary Curtis
Cover designed by Hilary Glanville

© Health Education Authority, 1992
First printed May 1992

British Library Cataloguing-in-Publication Data.
A catalogue record for this book is available from the British Library.

ISBN 0 7279 0745 X

Published by:

British Medical Association Foundation for AIDS
BMA House
Tavistock Square
London WC1H 9JP

Printed by:

Chameleon Press Limited
5-25 Burr Road
London SW18 4SG

To the memory of John Dawson.

Introduction

Hilary Curtis
Executive Director,
British Medical Association Foundation for AIDS,
London

This book is the product of the Second International Workshop on Prevention of Sexual Transmission of HIV and other Sexually Transmitted Diseases, a multidisciplinary workshop held jointly by the UK Health Education Authority and the British Medical Association Foundation for AIDS in Cambridge in March 1991.

Co-sponsored by the World Health Organisation (WHO) and held under the auspices of Mrs Catherine Lalumière, Secretary General of the Council of Europe, the "Promoting Sexual Health" workshop attracted about 200 invited experts who included health promotion and health education specialists from statutory and voluntary sector agencies and academic institutions. It focussed especially on sexual health promotion within the European context, with most participants coming from this region including the countries of central and Eastern Europe. In this respect it differed slightly from the First International Workshop, held by the Dutch Foundation for STD Control in 1989, which was inter-regional but with an emphasis on the developed world and of which the published proceedings[1] have become a standard text on the subject.

Sexual Health and Health Promotion

Between the first and second workshops there were substantial advances in linking HIV and AIDS prevention programmes into wider strategies directed towards STDs prevention, family planning and reproductive health, and general promotion of healthy, fulfilling and responsible patterns of sexual behaviour. For example, in the UK the Health Education Authority had adopted "HIV, AIDS and Sexual Health" as the official title of its programme, while in the voluntary sector the Terrence Higgins Trust had collaborated with Group B, a long-standing but previously not widely known support group for gay men with hepatitis B, to develop new health education materials promoting hepatitis B immunisation while reinforcing messages about HIV and safer sex. At the international level, too, WHO was integrating its Global Programme on AIDS with that on STDs.

These developments largely reflected the consensus of expert opinion and the first workshop's conclusions. When one considers that HIV is only the most serious of a range of sexually transmissible agents including several viruses which are as yet incurable, and that even curable infections such as gonorrhoea, chlamydia and syphilis continue to take their toll of pain, infertility and human misery, it is apparent that the significance of sexual behaviour for the public health extends well beyond prevention of AIDS, and that purely treatment-oriented approaches hold no solution to the problem. However, as this book describes, integration of HIV prevention with control of STDs is not entirely without pitfalls. Several factors necessitate a careful and considered approach, such as that behaviours considered "low risk" for HIV may still transmit other STDs; that people have widely different attitudes to and perceptions of different diseases; and that the relative benefits and drawbacks of primary prevention through behaviour change and secondary prevention through screening, case-finding, contact tracing and treatment differ substantially for curable and non-curable conditions.

There have also been developments in thinking about the scope and principles of health promotion, and in particular its relation to health education. Education, to inform people about health risks and how these can be prevented and to develop individuals' skills in making and implementing behavioural choices, plays an essential role in promoting health, whether in the context of tobacco, alcohol and other drugs, accident prevention, diet and physical exercise, or sex. But effective health promotion encompasses much more than just education directed at the individual level. The limitations of the individual approach as a model for health promotion are particularly apparent when considering marginalised or disadvantaged groups within society, who may be least in control of their own lives and least able to respond to information or exhortation.

The Ottawa Charter for Health Promotion[2] identifies five key elements: building healthy public policy; creating supportive environments; strengthening community action; developing personal skills; and reorienting services. The organisers of the "Promoting Sexual Health" workshop made a conscious effort, in briefing speakers, participants and rapporteurs, to ensure that these wider aspects of health promotion were thoroughly addressed.

The Format of the Workshop

The specific objectives of the "Promoting Sexual Health" workshop were:

- To share information and experience, and review progress in the prevention and control of the sexual transmission of HIV and other STDs;

- To develop a broadly based framework for promoting sexual health, and to identify practical measures to improve linkages between HIV/STD prevention and other health education/health promotion programmes;

- To consider, in particular, the effects of current socio-political changes in Europe on the organisation and impact of sexual health education/health promotion programmes;

- To recommend strategies for overcoming barriers in implementation of effective sexual health programmes (including HIV/STD prevention) with particular emphasis on:

     Building healthy public policy;
     Creating supportive environments;
     Strengthening community action;
     Developing personal skills;
     Reorienting services.

Like the first workshop, the meeting included plenary addresses from internationally recognised speakers (most of whom took the opportunity to participate throughout the workshop) together with interdisciplinary working groups which met repeatedly over a period totalling several hours. The working groups covered target audiences for health promotion measures (eg young people, women, men who have sex with men) and contexts or subject areas (eg family planning and reproductive health, condoms promotion, and the political and legislative framework for sexual health promotion).

In addition, as an experimental measure, some short informal discussion sessions were timetabled at the meeting on the themes of: bridge-building, integration and normalisation – always a good thing?; uncertainty and conflicting messages in health education – how much do they matter?; the impact of global and regional political change; AIDS, the media and the moral minority; and community organisations and peer group education. Although these discussions were not formally recorded, they provided an opportunity for cross-fertilisation between participants in different working groups as, in many cases, the themes were relevant to health promotion for several target audiences and in a variety of contexts. During the meeting there was also a display of health education materials from the various countries represented, and this exhibition and the workshop social events provided further occasions for informal interaction.

Prior to the meeting participants received a programme booklet which included abstracts of the plenary papers and reports from several European countries describing the local epidemiology of HIV and STDs, the structure of health promotion services and preventive strategies undertaken, and the broad legal and cultural context within the country concerned. In addition a background paper was prepared for each working group to introduce the specific issues affecting the relevant target audience or context for health promotion. Thus the scene was set for high-level, intensive discussion of strategies for sexual health promotion in the Europe of the 1990s.

Following the meeting, copies of the background papers for each working group and transcripts of the closing plenary session, in which brief reports were presented by each group, were circulated to all participants. Subsequently the recommendations and conclusions which the groups had included in these reports were condensed together into a booklet which was distributed widely to participants and others with an interest in sexual health promotion strategies and policy development. These summary conclusions and recommendations are reproduced in Appendix 1 (see page 173).

This Book

The plenary papers and fuller, written reports from the working groups are contained within this volume. Multi-author works such as conference proceedings sometimes attract criticism from reviewers for being uneven and lacking an overall, unified message. It is true that this work reflects a diversity of viewpoints and is varied in style and content. But when dealing with a subject as rich and complex as health promotion, variety can be a strength. Moreover, despite the different ideas and approaches reflected within this book, certain powerful and coherent themes emerge:

- The first, perhaps most forcefully expressed by Ekeid (see page 8), is that sexuality and its physical expression are positive, enjoyable, valuable and essential elements of human nature, and that concerns about adverse consequences of sexual activity must not be allowed to overshadow this fact.

- Secondly, it is not enough to look at the behaviour of individuals in isolation — a theme developed in various ways in several chapters. Effective sexual health promotion entails not only education for individuals to furnish them with the knowledge and skills to choose healthy lifestyles, but also wider interventions to build supportive public policies and social environments, to strengthen communities' ability to respond, and to re-orient services in more accessible and "user-friendly" ways, with particular attention to the needs of vulnerable and marginalised groups within society.

- Health education about HIV/AIDS and STDs takes two forms, and both are needed simultaneously. One is education *targetted* towards specific population groups according to their needs, and this involves a variety of techniques including outreach, peer-led, and community development approaches. The other is *diffuse* or *broad-brush* education, directed largely through the mass media, in order to maintain HIV/AIDS and sexual health issues on the public agenda, to influence the climate of social opinion and to reach some individuals who are at risk of infection but are not reached by targetted methods because they do not identify sufficiently closely with any of the specific groups concerned.

These themes, and others, are developed within the book, along with many examples of successful and not-so-successful projects from different countries. Nevertheless, the limited time available at the workshop has meant that certain topics were not covered in as much depth as one might like. For example, the importance of STD clinics as a setting for health promotion, through one-to-one counselling and education by health advisers or other methods, received only limited attention and could usefully be explored in greater depth in future meetings. Also, some working groups, faced with the immense challenge of HIV/AIDS prevention, found it difficult to expand their discussions fully to cover the wider questions posed by other STDs. It is perhaps a measure of the scale and complexity of the issues involved that this book is only a stage along the way to a comprehensive vision of sexual health promotion for the 1990s and beyond.

In editing these proceedings, I have tried to retain the vigour, the excitement and the imagination which was present at the workshop. I am grateful to the Health Education Authority, the Commission of the European Communities and the British Medical Association Foundation for AIDS for making their publication and distribution possible. Although much is lost in the transition to paper, the organisers and co-sponsors hope that this book will enable a much wider readership to share the fruits of the workshop and will provide a challenge and stimulus to all involved in promoting sexual health.

References

1. Paalman M (ed). Promoting safer sex. Amsterdam/Lisse: Swets & Zeitlinger, 1990.

2. World Health Organisation. Ottawa Charter for Health Promotion. Copenhagen/Geneva: WHO, 1986.

Opening Statements

Sir Donald Acheson KBE FRCP FRCS FFPHM FFOM
Chief Medical Officer
Department of Health
London

Thank you for giving me the opportunity to come to this workshop on promoting sexual health. I would like to add my welcome on behalf of the Department of Health, and to thank the co-sponsors, WHO's Global Programme on AIDS and the Health Education Authority who are partners with us in the Department of Health in the fight against the spread against HIV. I also thank the BMA Foundation for AIDS, which is a co-sponsor, and the many other non-governmental organisations, including for example, the National AIDS Trust, who are also represented here for their work and support over many years.

The topic of this workshop comes at a crucial moment, because the early successes which we have had in our efforts to educate and to change behaviour towards safer sex have recently suffered at least one significant setback. This a moment for reappraisal or at least reinforcement of the messages.

1991 is close to the tenth anniversary of the definition of AIDS, and it is perhaps fifteen to twenty years since the silent escalation of the spread of HIV began. We were not certain ten years ago, but we are certain now, that HIV is primarily and predominantly a sexually transmitted disease. And we are also certain now that, globally speaking, the predominant means of transmission is vaginal intercourse. The other types of transmission, through blood transfusion, factor VIII, intravenous drug abuse and nosocomial spread, are unwelcome secondary methods of transmission which are associated with modern medical technology and its abuse.

Globally, over the last ten years, the pandemic has continued to develop and spread rapidly. If I were to pick out some of the most unfavourable trends over the last year or two, they would include: the spread of the high prevalence in some sub-Saharan Africa countries from urban to rural neighbourhoods; the spread within intravenous drug abuse populations and prostitute populations in South-East Asia; heterosexual spread in South America and the Caribbean; the increasingly high rates within the urban poor in cities in the United States; and the high prevalence in intravenous drug abusers along the Mediterranean littoral where so many people from this country go for their holidays.

During the ten year period the work of all of you here has introduced a measure of candour about sex which I sincerely hope is irreversible. Also, I have no doubt at all that the efforts of those present have resulted in many thousands, perhaps tens of thousands of people not becoming infected who would otherwise have been infected. But there remains, and this is really my first point, an extraordinary ignorance about sexual behaviour almost everywhere, so that in most places we have no baseline against which we can measure progress and change towards sexual health.

The second point I want to make is an obvious one. It is that the key to controlling the spread of HIV lies in our knowledge of the determinants of the transmission of the virus from infected to non-infected. In respect of sexual transmission, the link with the presence of other sexually transmitted diseases which cause inflammation of the genital tract is now beyond question. We know that not only ulcerative conditions, like syphilis, chancroid and herpes, but other inflammatory conditions of both male and female genital tracts, including gonorrhoea, chlamydia and trichomonas, help the virus to be transmitted from a person who is infected.

But that is not the only link with sexually transmitted diseases, because HIV itself may delay the healing of ulcers in the genital tract, and also aggravate the course of both syphilis and gonorrhoea. So perhaps the most important single factor which influences the spread of HIV, as the result of sexual intercourse, is the presence of other inflammatory conditions of the genital tract. In addition we know that gender is important. The risk of transmission from men to women is greater by a factor two than that from women to men, and an approximately similar relative risk exists between penetrative anal intercourse and penetrative vaginal intercourse.

The issue of circumcision is more complicated, and I do not want to enter in any detail an area which is to some extent controversial. But I am impressed with the probable importance of sub-preputial hygiene and the fact that the uncircumcised man with poor hygiene is more inclined to the inflammatory condition balanitis than the circumcised. I was fascinated to read a leader in the New England Journal of Medicine[1] which was arguing, I suspect correctly, against routine circumcision for hygienic reasons. But the following quotation seemed to me to be a little impractical: "At puberty, boys should be instructed to clean under the foreskin as part of each bath or shower". Having recently visited the brothels in Bombay, I didn't notice any water, let alone soap, and I wonder how many boys who approach puberty in the world have an opportunity to bath frequently.

More work needs to be done in the matter of the factors which influence transmission. But we already know enough to see that HIV spread and its control must be part of a wider campaign which brings into focus the whole area of sexually transmitted disease.

The past ten years have seen a number of important successes in our efforts towards better sexual health. In spite of cynicism about the feasibility of changing sexual behaviour, there has been a quite astonishing reduction in risky behaviour amongst gay men in most of the world. This includes reduction in penetrative anal intercourse, and in number of partners, and an increase in use of condoms. In some countries following these changes rectal gonorrhoea almost disappeared. There was even greater cynicism about the possibility of changes in behaviour in intravenous drug abusers, but nevertheless quite striking progress has been made, and in many parts of the world there has been a marked reduction in sharing of equipment. In both situations it has been possible to show reduction in rates of transmission of HIV. In women, in many countries of Europe at any rate, there was already a downward trend in gonorrhoea and this continued and in some places the decline became steeper. In Britain since 1986, there has been an increase in the sales of condoms of about 30%. A sharp increase occurred after the original campaign early in 1987. Sales have gradually increased further at the rate of about 3% per annum.

But in the last year or two there has unfortunately been definite evidence that, in respect of gay men, there has been a return of rectal gonorrhoea, together with an upturn in the trend in gonorrhoea throughout the United Kingdom, in The Netherlands, in Australia and in Canada. This is discouraging. It gives us two lessons to take away: one is the need further to help gay men and others at risk to sustain a change in behaviour; but secondly, there is a wider inference we should draw, and that is that we should look more seriously at obtaining permanent changes in behaviour in the middle term by investing much more effort in the schools. We have to face up to the political difficulties not only in respect of sex education itself, but in introducing the issues of heterosexuality and homosexuality in younger people than is currently the case.

But in spite of this setback we should keep the matter in proportion, because as I have said before I have no doubt at all that, due to the efforts of those present and others, many people who would otherwise been infected with HIV continue to avoid the infection. It is apparent to all of us that sexually transmitted diseases are social diseases and HIV is no exception. From time immemorial, sexually transmitted disease has flourished most of all among the urban poor, where poverty is complicated by overcrowding and family breakdown leads to social disintegration. Cities in many parts of the world are characterised by large populations of transient males, migrant labourers, truck drivers, railway workers, commercial travellers, people labelled as foreigners, and, at the seaports, sailors. In cities, there are also often large pools of unsupported young women who, for economic reasons, have to sell sex for food and the necessities of life. Also, today we have the added complication, which wasn't present in the nineteenth century, of the perversion of science by the production of designer drugs such as crack, and the misuse of mass-produced plastic syringes.

It seems to me that, short of a generally available one shot vaccine or a fully effective antimicrobial agent for which we must all continue to hope, it will be necessary for us to address the underlying social issues if we are to make progress, and in particular the problems of impoverished illiterate and exploited women. We will have to go wider even than programmes to control inflammatory diseases of the genital tract. Information about HIV and its prevention will need to be integrated into general education and also into family planning and mother and baby programmes. There will also need to be campaigns against illiteracy and help for women to gain more control over their lives and their bodies.

References

1. Poland R L. The question of routine neonatal circumcision. N Eng J Med 1990; **322**: 1312-15.

Dr Svein-Erik Ekeid MB BS MA
Regional Coordinator,
World Health Organisation Global Programme on AIDS,
WHO Regional Office for Europe,
Copenhagen

Mr Chairman, Colleagues and Friends, ·

The emergence of the HIV/AIDS pandemic has renewed interest in the right to sexual health and a fulfilling sexual life for everyone, and in promoting safe sexual practices for everyone regardless of sexual life, regardless of sexual orientation and lifestyle. The success of the first international workshop on preventing the sexual transmission of HIV and other STDs, *Promoting Safer Sex*, organised by the Dutch Foundation for STD Control in 1989 bears witness to that, as does your presence here today at the second workshop, *Promoting Sexual Health*.

Worldwide, it is estimated that sexual intercourse accounts for some 80% of the total cases of HIV transmission so far. In Europe about 40% of the cumulative total of AIDS cases have been in people infected through anal or vaginal sexual intercourse, and indications are that sexual transmission is increasing at a relatively much faster rate than other forms of transmission.

In Europe at present, heterosexual transmission is increasing particularly sharply, and it may be useful to remind each other what this means in the European setting: it means there is heterosexual transmission from men to women, but that relatively speaking very little heterosexual transmission is taking place in the other direction at the moment. Whether this state of affairs will continue will no doubt be an item of discussion during this workshop.

There are indications that sexual transmission between men is again increasing in some groups and in some countries in Europe at present. No doubt the whys, wherefores and possible solutions will be discussed here as well.

Injecting drug users as a group remain very much at risk of HIV infection in Europe. It is important to remember that the sexual behaviour of drug users and their partners is likely to determine the future growth of the HIV pandemic in European countries. This is not least important in relation to possible developments in the countries of Central and Eastern Europe.

However, having said this, I think it might be pertinent to warn against self-fulfilling prophecies of doom. In our efforts to be proactive, we must not pave the way for the pandemic. The situation in Eastern Europe is of particular concern for two reasons:

- The development of the epidemic is so far five years behind the rest of Europe, which has given us an opportunity to intensify prevention efforts which we must not miss; however

- The other common feature is that the countries in question, generally speaking, lack human, technical and financial resources to implement these efforts. This is particularly so in the field of health promotion. The assistance and support of other European member states with greater experience of this particular problem and more abundant financial abilities are, therefore, vital to their HIV/AIDS prevention and control programmes.

This is neither the time nor the place for a detailed discussion of the initiative launched by the Global Programme on AIDS, Regional Office for Europe, towards supporting the countries of Central and Eastern Europe in their national programmes of HIV/AIDS prevention and control. It is sufficient today to remind you of the slogan for

World AIDS Day 1991: *Sharing the Challenge.*

In the words of the Director General of WHO, Dr Nakajima:

> "... *no country can combat the disease in isolation. Preventing the spread of HIV, caring for those affected, and minimising the social and economic repercussions of the AIDS pandemic require the strength that comes from partnership.*"

HIV is transmitted through sexual and other behaviours that are intimate, taboo, or even denied. In efforts to promote sexual health there is a need officially and explicitly to recognise that sexuality is mainly a recreational activity, not only a procreational activity. We need to see sexual health in its broadest spectrum, where reproductive health is an important aspect but not the sole point of interest, and where STDs and HIV (however seriously they threaten enjoyment, health and life) represent the small, negative side of the equation. In this sense their importance lies in the threat they pose to joy, infatuation, love, expression of feelings, and needs for bodily contact.

I am sure you will not misunderstand my message. But let me make it quite clear. I do not denigrate the importance of STDs and HIV infection for the individual concerned or for society. On the contrary. However, we must not let problems of sexual health overshadow the joys of enjoying sexual health. That is the very reason for promoting sexual health in a positive sense. We must not be ensnared by religion or other ideologies into looking at sexuality as a problem. In all expressions, life and health will meet obstacles to their enjoyment. STDs and HIV infection *are* obstacles to sexual health and expressions of sexual life. However, solutions to the problems of HIV infection and other STDs must be founded on a basic belief in sexuality as a positive force, and the right to sexual health as a basic human right along the lines of the right to health in general.

We are all here because we believe in the positive and attractive aspects of sex and sexuality. However, all too often these aspects, at conferences like this one, fall under the shadow of preoccupation with the problematic aspects of sexuality and sexual health.

Let us commit ourselves, before turning to HIV infection and other STDs, to reconfirm our belief in sexuality as a great, a positive aspect of being human. Let us reconfirm the right of every individual, regardless of sexual orientation, to enjoy sex with another consenting adult. Let us praise sexual enjoyment in its many and varied pleasurable expressions. Let us recall that these are our commitments and firm beliefs, and that no adversity, including HIV/AIDS and other STDs, shall seduce us to think otherwise of this fundamental expression of human nature.

With this background, it is my pleasure to convey to you all, organisers and participants, the best wishes for a successful workshop that will give guidance and directives for our further efforts in the important field of promoting sexual health, from WHO's Regional Director for Europe, Dr Jo Asvall, and from Dr Mike Merson, Director of the Global Programme on AIDS.

Epidemiological Perspective: an Overview of HIV/STDs/Reproductive Health in Europe

Peter Piot
WHO Collaborating Centre on AIDS
Institute of Tropical Medicine,
Antwerp

I will discuss recent trends in STDs and HIV infection in Europe, but will not go into details about trends in HIV prevalence and incidence, as this was very well discussed by Noel Gill at the Lausanne meeting on Assessing Preventive Strategies.

First of all, I would like to acknowledge my colleagues from various European countries who provided data on STDs and HIV infection. It was striking that it is much easier to obtain data on HIV than on STDs. But it is critical not to neglect STDs both because of the problems they create in themselves, and also since they are risk factors for HIV transmission, and may provide good indicators of high risk behaviour.

In many cities in Europe there has been a spectacular decline in incidence in HIV infection and other STDs in homosexual men. For instance, in Amsterdam between 1981 and 1987 the incidence in a cohort of gay men had declined to zero for HIV infection, and nearly to zero for rectal gonorrhoea, and the incidence of gonorrhoea in gay men in general had decreased drastically by 1988[1].

All very good news, and people were quite optimistic about behavioural modification and the effects of health promotion. Similar trends were observed, in gay men at least, in syphilis and hepatitis B virus infection, which turned out to be one of the best indicators of behavioural change in this population. However, not all news on STDs in Europe is as reassuring, as will be shown below.

Conventional Bacterial STDs

Sweden has an impressive record of epidemiological surveillance of gonorrhoea with data going back as far as 1912. At the present moment, in Sweden at least, there is an all time historical low in the incidence of gonorrhoea, despite the fact that diagnostic possibilities in 1987 and 1991 are obviously much better developed than the beginning of the century[2]. This trend has been observed in all Western and North European countries. Gonorrhoea has now become a rare disease in several countries. It is also striking that the decline in the incidence of gonorrhoea in most Western European countries began before AIDS was ever heard of, or before AIDS control and prevention campaigns actually started.

This decline has been greatest in gay men. For instance, in England and Wales, the incidences of syphilis and gonorrhoea for adult men and adult women are approximately the same, whereas in the past both diseases were much more common in men. The closing of this gap is a result of the decline in incidence in men[3].

Also new and interesting is data from several countries, the best documented being from Amsterdam, that the proportion of repeaters, that is people who have a prior history of an STD, is increasing among those with gonorrhoea. For instance, in the Amsterdam STD clinics, the proportion of patients who were repeaters increased by about 50% over a period of five years. That indicates or suggests that a limited group of highly sexually active individuals continue to put themselves at risk for STDs: this group may become increasingly important in the epidemiology and spread of STDs, and probably of HIV as well[4].

Changing Perspectives in the Epidemiology of STDs

1. Development of improved diagnostic tests resulting in recognition of unexpectedly large reservoirs of incurable viral STDs (HSV, HPV, HIV).

2. Differentiation of risk factors from risk markers.

3. Growing emphasis on the importance of health care seeking behaviour for the incidence of bacterial STDs (as opposed to viral STDs).

4. Growing emphasis on primary prevention through behavioural change rather than on secondary prevention through diagnosis and treatment for control of viral STDs.

Traditionally, reported STD rates in Southern Europe have been much lower than in Western and Northern Europe. This is probably at least in part due to a higher degree of under-reporting. For instance, in Italy, the same trends as elsewhere can be observed for gonorrhoea in a surveillance system based on STD clinics between 1986 and 1988, but it is also clear that within one country there are different patterns. As sexual mixing patterns are not identical everywhere, among countries and within particular countries we may see epidemiological differences. Thus, in Northern and Central Italy there has been a marked decline in the incidence of gonorrhoea but this has not been observed in the Southern part of the country, although under-reporting is believed to be much more of a problem in the Southern part of Italy than in the other parts[5]. It is something we have to bear in mind; just as there is no standard pattern of AIDS in Africa or "African AIDS", there is no such thing as "European AIDS". There are multiple epidemics and even within a country, one may distinguish several types of epidemiology of HIV and STDs. I believe we need to adjust our interventions much more to that knowledge.

Chlamydia trachomatis infection has now become the most common and major bacterial sexually transmitted disease in Western and Northern Europe, and probably also in the rest of Europe. For a long time it was heavily under-estimated because of lack of diagnostic facilities. It is depressing that in many countries of our continent, which is among the richest parts of the world, diagnostic facilities for chlamydial infection are still not widely available. Sweden has been a leading country in chlamydia control programmes in Europe, and also Belgium, where diagnostic services were introduced early. The immediate result was a dramatic increase in the number of people found to be infected with chlamydia, particularly amongst women since we focussed our efforts on them. In Belgium we have not seen yet a decline in the number of cases[6] but in Sweden, probably as a result of increased diagnostic activity for chlamydial infection, the number of diagnosed cases is now slowly declining.

There are very few epidemiological data on the complications of STDs. These complications and sequelae are particularly disturbing for women, and they are the major reason for trying to control STDs. Data on salpingitis, on ectopic pregnancy, on infertility, are available but most of the time hidden somewhere in a morass of other health indicators and data. Sweden again has the best data. Between 1970-1974 and 1980-1984 there was a marked decline in the number of cases of salpingitis, but particularly of the proportion of cases due to gonococcal infection. About 20 years ago, one salpingitis case out of four was due to gonorrhoea compared to only about 10% now[2]. *C. trachomatis* is now the leading cause of salpingitis in Europe. There is clearly a need for more data in more countries.

So far the good news, now what about the bad news? Firstly, in the US and in some European cities, there has been an increase in gonorrhoea, particularly in gay men and particularly of rectal gonorrhoea. Thus in Seattle in North-West USA there was an increase of such cases. Similar results have been observed in Amsterdam, Australia and in the UK, and this is of course very disturbing. It is also occurring in smaller cities[4]. For instance in Leeds in the UK, there was a decline of gonorrhoea over the years and a decline of the percentage of cases in homosexual men down to 2-3% of total cases, but last year 12% of the cases of gonorrhoea were in homosexual men[7]. This is back to the figures of the beginning of the decade.

It is not very clear who these men are, and what it all means. It is striking that we do not know exactly what rectal gonorrhoea means as an indicator of sexual practices. A recent survey from London reported that about half of the men with rectal gonorrhoea claimed to have had anal intercourse with a condom or had no receptive

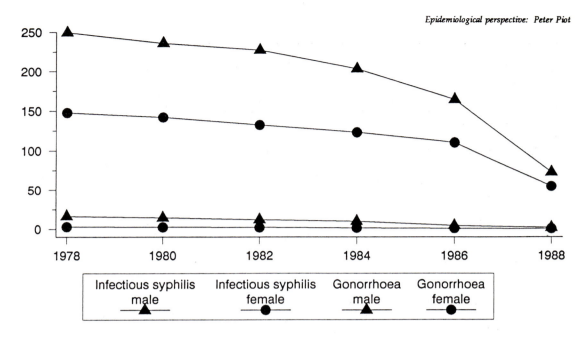

Figure 1: Rates of gonorrhoea and syphilis per 100,000 population aged 15-59 years, England and Wales.

Source: Ref 3

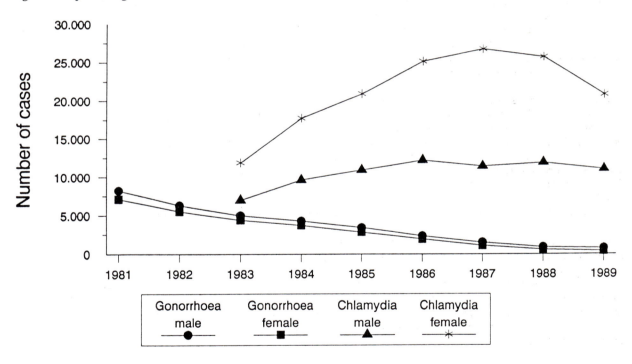

Figure 2: Laboratory reports on chlamydial and gonococcal infections in Sweden.

Source: Statens Bakteriol. Laborat., Stockholm

anal intercourse at all. It may be that so-called safe, or relatively safe, sexual practices can transmit infections such as gonorrhoea[8].

These very recent observations need confirmation, before we can tell whether the rise in incidence is sustained, whether we see a levelling off or whether this increase will continue. But it raises the question of whether this data reflects a failure of our efforts to modify behavioural risks for STDs after nearly ten years of success. The

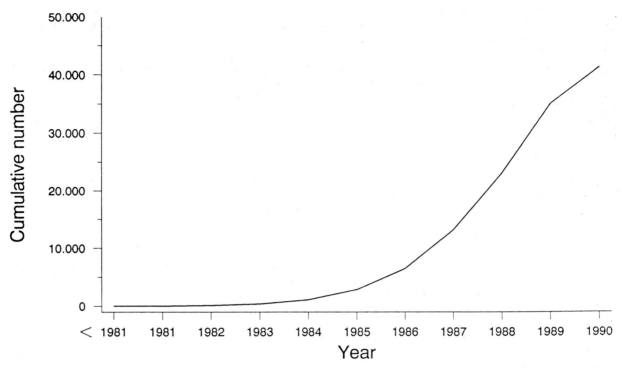

Figure 3: Cumulative AIDS cases in 32 European countries

Source: *Eur. Centre Epidemiol. Mon. AIDS*

reasons for these changes are not clear and are probably multiple. But it seems unlikely that the data result from improved surveillance of STDs in recent years, since they were first reported in populations with a strong tradition of STD services and surveillance.

It seems that the rising STD trends reflect a failure to sustain behavioural change by homosexual men, and that there may be two phenomena occurring simultaneously. Firstly, it is striking from the US data that a large proportion of gay men with an STD are very young, reflecting the entry of younger, possibly less cautious men into the homosexual population. Many of these men were not sexually active in the early 80's when the traumatic recognition of a new life-threatening STD infection contributed considerably to the behavioural change in homosexual men. However, and secondly, the data show that most homosexual men with an STD are older, suggesting that so-called behavioural "relapse" is occurring as well. Knowing the reasons for this "relapse" is extremely important for the further development of health promotion strategies. We have the crude figures and now we have to find out, by more detailed studies, what is really going on, who are these people, and why is this occurring.

Trends in Viral STDs

Increasing numbers of cases of other viral infections are seen in STD clinics. Briefly and in general, STD clinics in Europe are overflowing with people with genital warts, human papilloma virus infection, and with herpes infection. This is a tremendous problem because we have no really good treatment and control strategies, we do not know what to do. It is reflected in an increase in the incidence of cervical cancer virtually all over Europe. The trend may be partially due to better and earlier recognition of human papilloma virus and cervical cancer; but it is probably the result of further spread of this virus in the population.

Now, turning to AIDS, the news is mixed, some bad, some good. The cumulative number of AIDS cases in 32 European countries as reported by the European centre for epidemiological monitoring of AIDS in Paris, is now rapidly approaching 50,000 cases[9]. The picture varies from country to country according to transmission groups, and I will just draw your attention to the extremes: in The Netherlands the overwhelming majority of cases is in homosexual men and it continues that way; in Spain and Italy drug users are making up the majority of the cases; in Belgium there is a large proportion of heterosexuals; and in Romania transmission through blood products is a major mode of spread.

What are the trends? The first trend is that more women are acquiring HIV infection and are getting AIDS, and these women are on average younger than men who have AIDS. In West Germany the proportion of women among AIDS cases has increased from 5% to 10% by the end of last year[10].

Secondly, a greater proportion of people developing AIDS now were known to be HIV positive before the diagnosis of AIDS than used to be the case. This is important in terms of opportunities for intervention, as anti-retroviral chemotherapy will become more and more available in the near future.

The third trend is that while HIV prevalence rates have become established in the larger centres, there has also been spread to smaller centres as suggested by data from the UK, for HIV prevalence in London and outside London. The trend is for the two to come closer and closer to each other. This has also been observed in France and Germany.

Finally as a trend in Europe, since last year intravenous drug users are now accounting for nearly as many cases of AIDS as homosexual men. This is particularly the case in Southern Europe. This does not mean the absolute number has decreased among homosexual men, only the proportion of the total number of patients with AIDS. In addition, particularly in Amsterdam and in Italy, studies indicate that unsafe sexual behaviour is very common among IV drug users and so this is an additional source for sexual spread of HIV infection in the population[11].

Conclusions

Finally, where are we going? Firstly, at least in Europe, demographics are on our side. We do not expect a large increase in the population between 15 and 40 years old that is potentially the most exposed to sexually transmitted infections in our areas, except for migrant populations. On the other hand, in the developing world there is only bad news from the perspective of demographics and sexually transmitted diseases. Projections made by the European Centre on AIDS in Paris, using four or five different models to produce short term projections for 1989-1992, show an incredibly wide range of possibilities. So we really do not know what to expect, particularly in view of the changes in Eastern Europe and Central Europe, and the fact that we lack a clear picture of what is happening in the heterosexual population and the IV drug using population.

What are the recent trends in STDs within Europe?

- There is an overall decline in bacterial STDs, but an increase in patient visits for viral STDs, particularly human papilloma virus infections and genital warts.

- There is an increase or stabilisation of chlamydial infection in most countries, due to better and improved diagnosis.

- There are recent increases in incidence of rectal gonorrhoea in men and, in some countries, also of syphilis in heterosexuals, particularly in the major cities.

As far as HIV is concerned:

- There is much more rapid spread among IV drug users, who have become the largest group with HIV infection in Europe.

- There is a stabilisation amongst homosexual men, but a shift to younger men and also perhaps a rebound of infection in several cities now.

- Women make up an increasing proportion of people with HIV or AIDS, and the infection has spread to smaller cities.

In terms of conclusions I would like to mention four points:

- Firstly, epidemiological surveillance is useful, and we should use it. However, what is not clear is what type of surveillance is really useful, what is really needed. Do we sometimes put too much emphasis on trying to define, up to the last digit, the prevalence rates in a given population and this at high costs? What degree of precision do we need?

- It is discouraging that not much is done with data which comes out of surveillance programmes. What should we do with this data? How promptly should we react to small but significant increases, like increases in incidence of infections within small populations of gay men? Should we react to this, re-target our interventions on the basis of this data? The messages are sometimes confusing and we need more studies on the actual use of the data.

- There is a need for improved data on complications of STDs particularly in women, and on how well data on STDs reflects sexual behaviour.

- Finally, while trying to collect data on STDs in our region, I became even more convinced of the urgent need for coordination of STD surveillance data at European level, as has been done for AIDS. With the addition of public health to the basic treaty of the European Community, such an initiative should be politically feasible.

References

1. Van de Laar M J W, Pickering J, van den Hoek J A R, van Griensven G J P, Coutinho R A, van de Water H P A. Declining gonorrhoea rates in The Netherlands, 1976-88: consequences for the AIDS epidemic. Genitourin Med 1990; **66**: 148-155.

2. Kamwendo F, Forslin L, Danielsson D. Epidemiology and ætiology of acute non-tuberculous salpingitis. A comparison between the early 1970s and the early 1980s with special reference to gonorrhoea and use of intrauterine contraceptive device. Genitourin Med 1990; **66**: 324-329.

3. Catchpole M A. Sexually transmitted diseases: England and Wales, 1978-1990. Report. London: PHLS Communicable Disease Surveillance Centre, 1990.

4. Van den Hoek J A R, van Griensven G J P, Coutinho R A. Increase in unsafe homosexual behaviour. Lancet 1990; **336**: 179-180.

5. Greco D, Giulani M, Suligoi B, Panatta M, Giannetti A. Sexually transmitted diseases in Italy: clinical returns versus statutory notifications. Genitourin Med 1990; **66**: 383-386.

6. Walckiers D, Piot P, Stroobant A, Van der Veken J, Declerq E. Declining trends in some sexually transmitted diseases in Belgium. Genitourin Med 1991; **67**: 374-377.

7. Waugh M A. Resurgent gonorrhoea in homosexual men. Lancet 1991; **337**: 375.

8. Tomlinson D, French P D, Harris J R W, Mercey D E. Does rectal gonorrhoea reflect unsafe sex? Lancet 1991; **337**: 501-502.

9. European Centre for the Epidemiological Monitoring of AIDS. AIDS surveillance in the European Community. Paris: European Centre for the Epidemiological Monitoriing of AIDS, September 1991.

10. Koch M A, Bunikowski R, Esterman J, Pfeifer R, Schwardtländer B. AIDS und HIV in der Bundesrepublik Deutschland. München MMV: Medizin-Verlag, 1990, 153.

11. Van den Hoek J A R, van Haastrecht H J A, Scheeringa-Traast B et al. HIV infection and STD in drug addicted prostitutes in Amsterdam: potential for heterosexual HIV transmission. Genitourin Med 1989; **65**: 146-150.

Policy Perspective: a Comparison of National Programmes and Policies in Europe

Svein-Erik Ekeid
Regional Coordinator,
World Health Organisation Global Programme on AIDS,
WHO Regional Office for Europe,
Copenhagen

Overview and History of National Programmes

In 1989 the WHO Global Programme on AIDS, Regional Office for Europe, conducted a survey of AIDS policies and programmes in the European Region. The survey was updated in 1990. The responses from national programme managers in most cases also discuss the relations between the HIV/AIDS prevention and control programme in each country and the STD programme of that country and form the basis of much of this presentation.

For all 31 European member states it is fair to say that their national programmes for HIV/AIDS prevention and control are characterised by being vertical and self-contained. By "vertical" I mean that they are run top-down, with only limited concern for what is happening at the same time in other health service sectors.

The main explanation for the development of vertical HIV/AIDS programmes in the early stages of the epidemic in Europe may lie in the concern at that time for safeguarding of blood supplies. In most European countries there was great professional and public pressure for an immediate end to transmission by blood and blood products. In some countries, most usually due to pressure from gay organisations and not to foresight on the part of the public health authorities, a concurrent effort was started to promote prevention of sexual transmission of HIV, targetted particularly at men who have sex with men.

It can also be safely said that, in countries where politicians took an early and positive interest in concerted action, development of HIV/AIDS prevention and control programmes happened faster. In countries where the political leadership tended to deny or be complacent about the problems, much less comprehensive programmes developed, and took longer to find their feet as self-contained programmes. Comparative assessments of European HIV/AIDS prevention and control programmes also conclude that in most cases the successful launch of HIV/AIDS programmes was, in the early stages, often dependent on a high public health official in the country taking a strong and charismatic lead in overcoming public and political reluctance or complacency.

This is history, and as you are well aware, the force of the pandemic meant an expansion of vertical national programmes in all countries in Europe to encompass prevention of spread of HIV by the sexual routes, by illicit injection practices and through vertical transmission.

It is reasonable to conclude, however, that with only one or two exceptions, there were few attempts at that time genuinely to integrate HIV prevention and STD prevention programmes, or to achieve horizontal integration into public health and primary health care. In the light of the urgency of the situation, and for reasons discussed below, this lack of integration in fact contributed greatly to the early efficacy of HIV/AIDS prevention and control programmes in those countries able to respond quickly, with sufficient resources, and with strong public health and health promotion leadership.

It is also true that, for the newer national programmes developed by countries in Central and Eastern Europe during the last twelve months, there may be concern for horizontal integration of HIV/AIDS prevention and control within these plans, but there have been few attempts at this stage of their development to achieve genuine integration with programmes for STD control.

The Development of STD Programmes

The impression one gains is that the reasons for the lack of concerted or integrated HIV/AIDS and STD programmes may lie mainly in the way STD programmes had developed over the last forty to fifty years in Europe.

For many reasons, good and bad, STD programmes had tended either to become "quickly in-quickly out" programmes, ie the approach was often based simply on diagnosis and treatment, with no questions asked, in order not to embarrass the patient (or perhaps the staff?). Or, in countries where STD programmes contained elements of counselling, an element of distrust had often developed between the services and their clients. Services were often perceived as moralising and old-fashioned in their attitude to developing and changing sexual attitudes and mores. A new generation, of younger and better educated clients than characterised earlier STD patients, demanded respect for and an acceptance of their lifestyle which often was alien to STD service providers. The providers of STD services all too often knew everything about microbiology and STD pathology, and little about human sexology. Far too frequently, they took no interest in eliciting a sexual history from the patient or in asking pertinent questions over and above asking for symptoms and examining for signs of disease.

Whether the potential users of special STD services were in fact right about this lack of congruence between clients and providers may, of course, be a bone of contention. The widespread *perception* of lack of congruence was important, however, when an urgent decision had to be taken, in setting up HIV/AIDS programmes, as to the acceptability of STD control programmes as a main agency for public and personal communication with groups and individuals identified as targets for these developing HIV/AIDS prevention and control activities.

The Development of HIV/AIDS Programmes: Social Marketing and Psychosocial Counselling

For many reasons, some discussed below, a biomedical strategy could not be adopted by the new HIV/AIDS prevention and control programmes. Instead, lack of adequate diagnostic methods in the early stages, and the continuing lack of curative treatment for HIV infection, have both led to an approach based upon social marketing of messages targetted to specific groups and to the general public, and psychosocial counselling as a preventive tool at the individual level.

It is perhaps remarkable that, when social marketing approaches had been attempted in the past in STD prevention campaigns, they had not been proved particularly successful in reducing incidence of, for instance, gonorrhoea. This lack of success was, in itself, one of the indicators used to conclude that STD services might not be sufficiently trusted as originators of information and education directed at groups targetted for HIV/AIDS information. However, when social marketing was used to promote safer sex and condom use in the context of HIV/AIDS, one effect was a sharp acceleration in the long-term downward trend of conventional STDs in those countries which had the capacity to monitor STD incidence and prevalence.

Analysing this different response, we can perhaps detect another reason for the continued separation of HIV/AIDS and STD prevention programmes. HIV infection is *another* STD, but *not just any other* STD. The personal and societal consequences of HIV infection, and of catching other STDs, are perceived as qualitatively different by the affected individual, by health services, and by society. Most individuals, and most public health service managers, regard HIV infection with greater "seriousness" because of the short and long term individual consequences, for perspectives for health, for length and for quality of life. It presents different and more serious social consequences, demands and needs for health and other services, and the individual and societal financial impact is of a different magnitude.

HIV/AIDS revealed an existential crisis in European lifestyles. HIV infection became a symbol and a carrier of the mythological "evil". The appearance of the pandemic was traumatic to post-modern European culture. What was needed was, therefore, an approach to health promotion which would influence and allay the anxiety created by the appearance of this new "evil". This explains the failure of anxiety-provoking strategies in health promotion, which seemed to lead only to denial and to compensatory risk-taking behaviour by individuals unable to cope with the trauma.

Health promotion strategies which could face the problem of working through the anxiety that HIV/AIDS provoked needed to acknowledge sexuality as a positive and healthy life force. Only an individual who has the strength to say "yes" to sexuality has the strength to say "no" to risky sexual behaviour — to make the choice. Only those strategies which accepted that elements of sexuality — for instance the giving and receiving of semen — have a strong unconscious symbolic value to the individual were found to be sustainable. Sexuality expresses a part of a human being's continual search for affirmation of being a full, lovable and compassionate person. The sexual life we indulge in mirrors our self-image.

Innovative approaches thus had to be developed, which would incorporate and lay stress on personal contact in communication between the information/education provider and the targetted person. Approaches needed to be culturally specific, and interventions demanded mobilisation of individuals and groups who were directly affected. All these are, of course, sound principles of health promotion.

Almost as a paradox, this also required a parallel approach which was all-embracing. That is, individuals and groups at risk had continually to be seen not only as men-who-have-sex-with-men or as injecting-drug-users, but equally as individuals forming part of the general public. This meant not seeing it as "them and us"; not defining the general public as the heterosexual part of the population. It was necessary to keep more than one thought at a time in one's mind. There had to be lateral thinking, and room for a new science of chaos with instability at every point.

The strategy required was to develop an orchestra of activities, where the various interventions, seen together, achieve a higher degree of effectiveness than their sum alone. It was necessary at the same time to create distance and closeness, very specifically targetted interventions within a general atmosphere of understanding of the issue. The mountain has had to come to Mohammed, when Mohammed has been reluctant to come to the mountain.

The Relation between STD Programmes and HIV/AIDS Programmes: Where can we go from here?

There have been many occasions in many member states when these new approaches of HIV/AIDS prevention and control have wrestled with the entrenched and familiar approaches of the existing STD programmes. It has been argued time and time again that, since the old STD programmes had curtailed STDs, these same approaches would stop the spread of HIV.

But I believe, and I think that most HIV/AIDS programme managers would agree, that the old STD programmes were not the only or the main key to the successful curtailment of STDs in Europe, and (as I have tried to illustrate) that HIV infection is in many ways fundamentally different to treatable, non-life-threatening STDs.

This said, however, there are lessons to be learned from STD control programmes for people working with HIV/AIDS. Some of these lessons, unfortunately, are of a negative character and teach us what *not* to do: that coercive measures are contraindicated; that contact tracing and partner notification must be done in cooperation with the affected person, and with proper respect for confidentiality and for the need for consent.

There are countries, albeit exceptions, that have developed a reasonable common approach for HIV/AIDS and STD prevention services, particularly in relation to services for young people. It is not surprising that these exceptions are based upon taking the best of HIV/AIDS prevention and control programmes, discharging the traditional thinking and ossified practices in established STD programmes, and retaining what is good and fits our new and present situation and thinking. In other words, being very much aware of the limitations both of a pure psychological approach as I have just outlined, and of the biomedical approach in its pure form, which I am sure I need not elaborate upon.

The final answer has not been found as to the best form of integration and cooperation between HIV/AIDS programmes and STD programmes, or between vertical programmes of these kinds and the horizontal approaches of public health, primary health care and community care services. In a sense, of course, the final answer will never be developed. During this workshop, however, we must hope to find indicators for future directions and development. It is important to agree on models of good practice and examples of successful intiatives that can give us guidance, both for new approaches in member states with some experience of the epidemic, and for countries with low prevalences hitherto and an evolving problem. For the time being, I personally am in no doubt that:

- HIV/AIDS prevention and STD control need to be integrated horizontally;
- HIV/AIDS prevention and STD control need to work synergetically together;
- *But*, HIV/AIDS prevention and control programmes, and STD programmes, need to be retained as vertical programmes, at least at central levels.

Only by retaining this vertical element can we be assured of being able to continue exploring the development of interventions and to implement point interventions in areas and towards groups and individuals that might otherwise be forgotten. Last but not least, continued verticalisation is needed to ensure as far as possible that complacency is combatted with the necessary vigour, regardless of whether that complacency is among politicians who think the problem is solved, or among individuals striving to have a fulfilling and healthy sexual life in a world where the right and healthy choices are not always the easiest choices.

Finally, this is our task. As in all health promotion, so in promoting sexual health:

- Developing personal skills — empowerment;
- Strengthening community action;
- Creating supportive environments;
- Reorienting health and social services; and
- Building healthy public policies.

Only by developing HIV/AIDS prevention and control programmes, and STD control programmes, based on these principles can we achieve our aim:

- To make the *healthy* choices the *easy* choices as concerns our sexual life and sexual well-being.

5

Getting the Obvious to Stick: Linking Sexual Health/HIV/STDs to Global Issues of Poverty and Development

Tony Klouda
Coordinator,
AIDS Prevention Unit,
International Planned Parenthood Federation,
London

In the last four years I have been disturbed by the realities of much programming carried out by both expatriates and nationals in many villages and towns in the name of the prevention of the sexual transmission of HIV. Such programmes continue in large number, and I want to address myself to the issues raised by such programmes, rather than to the rhetoric that is often used to describe the programmes by their international supporters.

Definitions

In talking about global issues of poverty and development, it would be as well to start by saying how I will use these terms. Some may find this a bit simplistic, but I would like to talk of *poverty* as a relative lack of resources. By itself, such a concept is relatively useless, but it is when placed alongside four other clusters of disadvantage that we begin to get more of a feel for the political context, as these clusters can apply as much to economically disadvantaged as to sexual minorities. Different groups will have different balances of these clusters. These other clusters have been well described by Robert Chambers as:

- Physical weakness
- Vulnerability
- Isolation
- Powerlessness

As for *development*, I would like to talk of it as an *evolutionary process* in which people and societies adapt to new situations — by modifying either the situations or themselves. This approach to development will help us focus on two key features:

- That objectives in development are mostly related only to particular problems or situations as they arise, and are therefore changing constantly. There is a continuous cycle, or wheel, of development. This aspect gives development its political slant in terms of its balance between the disadvantaged, their advocates and the advantaged.

- That there is no country or group that can talk of themselves as either more or less developed than another, since each society develops in response to different situations. The particular new situation to which we are all developing is the presence of HIV.

Unlinking Poverty and AIDS

Before trying to link sexual health, HIV and STDs to global issues of poverty and development, let me do some unlinking first.*

We cannot blame poverty for AIDS. AIDS would exist even if poverty did not exist.

Much has been said about how poverty increases the impact of HIV infection and AIDS, and how it makes prevention harder. Thus there is no doubt at all about the following statements:

- That poverty at many levels can make the impact of AIDS worst on the poorest individuals and societies.

- That poor individuals and societies may find it harder to prevent AIDS or support people with HIV infection or with AIDS, due to their lack of resources, management and training (although it has been seen many times that poorer societies may mount more loving and caring responses than their richer counterparts).

- That the lack of resources in some societies still makes it very difficult to ensure some basic requirements such as an uninfected blood supply.

- That AIDS has been used as a reason for the continuance and maintenance of stigmatisation and prejudice concerning people and societies that are poor

- That AIDS has been used as an excuse for brutally increasing control of people who are poor or who are marginalised through isolation, jailing and assault.

In addition it is true that socio-economic inequality and poverty can lead to an increase in the sale of sex.

But all this seems to me very obvious, and I do not know that there is anything more to say about it. There is nothing particularly *new* that AIDS brings to the debate. We have known for millennia that with poverty lies ill-health and ill-a-whole-lot-of-other-things as well.

The social reformers at the end of the 19th century in Europe recognised this very well, and their social, legal and service reforms did more to change the face of health and improve the condition of people than any other public health or medical measure has done before or after.

There was nothing new about the impact of poverty when the Declaration was made at Alma Ata in 1978 on the need for all governments to develop appropriate Primary Health Care approaches in the context of political, social and economic change in order to ensure improved health for the poorest. "Health For All by the Year 2000" was the cry then, but it is hard to believe in that now.

There was nothing startling about the Black report in the UK in 1978 that drew forcible attention to the inequalities in health perpetuated by the policies of the UK government and that have yet to be addressed by it.

Despite this I continue to hear much talk about the inter-relationships of AIDS and poverty as though this *was* something of new or of particular interest.

Some have used the argument in a different way, and have suggested that AIDS forces us to look afresh at the social and economic inequalities that have always existed. At the dreadful infrastructures for health and social welfare in many countries. At the revolting and unjust way in which we hold many of the citizens of our own countries in traps of poverty from which they cannot escape. But these words often come from people who are *within* the "AIDS work set", and I do not think that AIDS itself has had any visible stimulus to national development programmes to deal with the issues of poverty in any new way. If we continue to mouth these platitudes with any expectation of success, we are deluding ourselves. If we wish to join forces with those who

---

* As this paper focuses on the issues of poverty, I will not be considering the development of people who do not suffer from the clusters of disadvantage, except in passing.

want to try to do something about socio-economic inequalities, then we should move out of programmes specifically aimed at prevention of the sexual transmission of HIV and integrate the work fully with programmes that *do* try to achieve such change. This would mean altering the objectives of the work.

Another reason for unlinking poverty from AIDS in this way is to clarify an incredibly simplistic approach to poverty that is now beginning to appear as the frustration grows amongst those who have taken on AIDS prevention in other countries as a job. This approach was expressed concisely in a recent letter to a British newspaper:

> *"The AIDS virus is spreading more rapidly than human institutions can respond to it. Charities such as Save the Children argue that it is by tackling poverty and inequality that HIV infection can be controlled in Third World countries.*
>
> *AIDS does indeed often begin among exploited and disadvantaged women who are forced to have many sexual partners. Certainly poverty plays a cruel role in spreading the infection, and all reasonable people want to see poverty alleviated.*
>
> *But it is common for HIV infection among prostitutes to double every 12 months or so, and it is fatuous to suppose that any organisation can make a dent in the social causes of prostitution in the next year or two. We must fight the war against AIDS as directly as possible, with the weapons we have — education, distribution of condoms, and vigorous treatment of sexually transmitted diseases. Pie-in-the-sky plans to tackle the spread of AIDS by relieving poverty are a cruel delusion that will lead to many otherwise avoidable deaths."*

This argument of course misses a fundamental point. Almost everyone would agree that education, distribution of condoms and treatment of sexually transmitted disease are a priority, and a large number of people are involved in doing just that. But I have not heard of anyone who has suggested a strategy to prevent AIDS that concentrates *only* on a vague commitment to *"tackling poverty"*. The fact is, try as people might, everyone has come unstuck with programmes of education, of condom promotion and of STD treatment when faced with the grim realities of some people's lives. And none of these programmes have achieved success with the poorest in timescales of less than *"12 months or so"*.

Development

This brings me to a more detailed look at the concept of development.

One thing we do know is that the mere provision of education, materials, resources or advice, whilst necessary, is not sufficient.

This lesson was learnt decades ago in Primary Health Care. We learnt that while the majority of most communities had the resources, education or supportive environments to benefit from the services offered by health, agricultural and educational ministries, a significant minority did not, and it was this minority that suffered the bulk of mortality and morbidity. This is the case in *any* community.

There are many examples that testify to the necessity but insufficiency of supply-side measures. A good example is the building of latrines. This often has little effect on overall health because oral-faecal disease continues in the children of the poorest families — who are left at home without adequate care whilst their (often single) parent works elsewhere. It is only with changes in labour relations and establishment of community care that such problems can be answered, but few communities have been able to do such things.

The situation is exactly the same when you consider the prevention of the sexual transmission of HIV. Take, for example, the fact that incidence of HIV infection amongst Hispanic and Black women in the Bronx is similar to the incidence of infection in women in Abidjan. The reasons for this are very much centred on the poverty or powerlessness of the women concerned in each of the communities. But one major point of difference (apart from the obvious political and cultural differences) is the fact that the women in the Bronx have had *theoretical* access to unlimited supplies of condoms, to treatment for STDs, and have been exposed to a great deal of educational and investigative effort.

Of course, this access is only illusory, since the situations of the women concerned deny them effective access to the STD treatment or to the condoms, and the education often does not start from their own perceptions of their own situation. There are examples from many parts of the world of similar situations in which power relations and economic control ultimately deny effective access of some people to crucial services. With the development of community-based organisations in the Bronx, this is changing, but this reinforces the point about the need for a developmental approach that coexists with improvements in the supply side. Unless this occurs, measures of increased condom sales, attitudinal change, and attendance at clinics will remain meaningless.

A further example of this lesson is provided by work with Nairobi sex workers where condom use has been increased, but HIV sero-prevalence continues to rise because of the failure to achieve condom use with all partners, the need to maintain constant effort with a group that is fluid in composition, and, of course, the failure of the condoms themselves.

Some people will point to the fact that even amongst groups that have no apparent disadvantage, and who have plenty of knowledge about sexual transmission of disease and have access to condoms and treatment for STDs, there is still sexual transmission of HIV. This seems to be true in Scandinavian countries where public discussion of sex and HIV have been carried out with relatively little embarrassment. There may be two points here.

- The first is that everyone will at some stage in their lives take some risk deliberately for a range of reasons, or in the heat of the moment. This simply cannot be avoided.

- The second is that experimentation with sex, especially for young people, can be excruciatingly difficult. How many of us can say we never have suppressed certain feelings or anxieties at the moment of sexual contact. I know very well that I have often been so anxious to negotiate any sex at all that negotiating *safer* sex was just one step too many.

These situations will continue to make it very difficult to achieve the *total* prevention of the sexual transmission of HIV. They affect everyone, whatever their advantage or disadvantage. We still do not know to what extent they determine the rate of spread of HIV or STDs, but since the incidence of HIV is greater in many (though not all) groups with the clusters of disadvantage, it would seem that our priority for the moment is to aim at the other limiting factors with these groups. Apart from the supply side, what does this mean in terms of development?

We are well used to hearing of the initiatives undertaken by groups on their own behalf in response to AIDS. Perhaps the most widely known are the various gay groups in the USA such as the Gay Men's Health Crisis, and the support groups for people with AIDS that have flowered in many countries such as the ones in Zambia or Uganda. There are many others who have achieved much both with their own HIV-positive groups and in advocacy to others.

Classically, as happened in the way other groups around the world have responded to a wide range of situations, the process in their development involved a sense of belonging to a community, together with their achieving agreement on an issue, a desire or a problem. The groups then acted together around that issue to change the situation or themselves — sometimes in conjunction with outsiders — and to form part of what we refer to rather trendily nowadays as supportive environments.

This, then, is successful evolutionary response to the stimulus of HIV infection. The next question is: is there any chance of helping other groups through the same process?

This is a crucial question, since there are often many problems when outside agencies try to initiate or become involved in this process. It can be hard for the outsiders to avoid setting the agenda of issues for the group of people involved. The outsiders themselves therefore represent a new situation to which people have to develop a response, and the response may well be one of a surface-obedient compliance. There follows a lot of activity and the trappings of change — posters are produced, groups are gathered and people are trained. Yet the fundamental issues (which affect *all* problems and not just AIDS) are often not addressed and so the problem continues.

Part of the setting of agendas is the preparation of "messages" which are essentially created by outsiders. People working in health promotion have known the problems inherent in this approach for decades, yet the lessons seemed to have been forgotten in many of the HIV and STD prevention campaigns that were mounted round the world.

results. This is why our UK Consortium of NGOs for AIDS Prevention in the Third World has concentrated so much on a development perspective that is integrated with other in-country development efforts, and on the strengthening of local institutions. These efforts, as I have said often, require time. But I can see no alternative to this if we are to achieve lasting results.

In the meantime, it is of course right to spend as much money as possible on ensuring that the basic supplies are in place, that information is provided, and that STDs can be treated locally. These things by themselves *will* have an impact for some people. It's just that we can't expect too much from their mere provision for the benefit of *all* people.

For all those used to the world of Primary Health Care, this is just a re-statement of the obvious. But then I live in the hope that one day we will really act on the obvious, and that the obvious will stick.

6

Building Links: Mutual Learning between AIDS and other Health Promotion Programmes

Rosmarie Erben
World Health Organisation,
Manila

The subject of this paper, *Building Links: Mutual learning between AIDS and other health promotion programmes*, is of vital importance for progress in health. In fact, it would be hard to find a health project of any worth which does not emphasize the need for coordination, in other words, for mutual learning and the building of links. Of course, the willingness to engage in mutual learning is a precondition for building links since linking requires understanding of each other's objectives, approaches and strategies. In turn, understanding implies the capacity to learn from each other, referring to what we see and hear, to what we feel and do ourselves.

The process of mutual learning leads to the notion of solidarity and rests on a common interpretation of the principles of health promotion. I have no doubt that all of us agree on what solidarity means in the field of HIV transmission and AIDS. However, do we all have a common perception of what health promotion stands for?

We often refer to the Ottawa Charter for Health Promotion[1], quote its basic principles and assume that its content is clear. Yet, in many instances, the concept of health promotion is reduced to one or the other of its elements. Often we focus on the development of personal skills or on community participation without taking into account the most important dimensions of health policies, cultural, social and ecological changes of society, and the creation of supportive environments. Even within WHO there are different interpretations of health promotion and we are still far from being able to state that the concept is clearly understood by all concerned.

Do we fully accept, for instance, that major aspects of health lie outside the health sector? Are we ready to abandon the medical model and to adopt the social model of health on which health promotion is based? This model is consumer-oriented, implies horizontal, multisectoral and multi-disciplinary approaches and therefore has many structural consequences. Are we equipped to cope with the day-to-day operational problems resulting from having a vast range of outside partners such as employers, trade unions, sickness funds, business groups, political parties, voluntary organisations and many others? And when we state that health has to be achieved through social and political processes, are we prepared to face the implications at the levels of planning and implementation?

The fact remains that the very strength of health promotion lies in its interdisciplinary nature and its broad approach to health problems, involving all sectors. Why is it, then, that the strategies often used in the prevention and control of HIV and AIDS focus on the psychological dimension of behaviour change?

One reason for this may be that sexual behaviour is seen as a purely personal matter, hence the focus on shaping sexual habits in the direction of safer sex. But past experience shows that such an approach is not sufficient. If we look at related fields such as smoking and alcohol consumption, we see that efforts at behavioural change must be integrated into a broad health promotion approach involving measures such as banning advertisements or cigarette machines and at creating, or increasing, smoke-free areas in public buildings and transport. There is no doubt that individual freedom to smoke and consume alcohol has to be respected. However, as soon as other people suffer from such behaviours, it becomes the responsibility of society and governments to take steps to protect the community as a whole.

The same is true with HIV transmission and AIDS. Sexual lifestyles are a private matter but measures are needed at the political level to foster supportive environments for responsible sexual behaviour.

There are other reasons for a reductionistic approach to health promotion. For instance, when we read the findings of the Glasgow survey on sex and AIDS among young people[2], we see that the respondents are aware of risks, know what to do to reduce these risks, but often are not acting accordingly. When confronted with these findings, our natural reaction is to turn to information, education, and communication as a means to overcome the problem. These are familiar strategies to us, and they are indeed most necessary and useful. But, as stated by Gerard Hastings from the University of Strathclyde in Scotland, who directed the survey, what is involved is in fact a cultural shift in our attitude to sex. This means not only tackling fundamental sexual issues, but also promoting coordinated action between schools, health services, employers, voluntary organisations, parents and the media. And when we come to free distribution of condoms, policy and legal aspects then head the list of planning items.

But let me come back now to the subject of my paper and discuss aspects of mutual learning between AIDS and other health promotion programmes. I have chosen young people and schools, the workplace, health services concerned with maternal and child health and with the transmission of sexual diseases, and the community. Then I will turn to experiences of personal health promotion in relation to chronic illness. What I will share with you are essentially reflections and questions. I am sure that the working groups will provide the workshop with concrete examples that will be precious in developing guidelines for action.

Young People and Schools

The peer approach represents one of the strategies that offers most to AIDS in learning from experience in other fields.

The use of peer leaders as facilitators for alcohol abuse prevention with adolescents, for instance, has been shown to be an essential component of successful programmes. The WHO collaborative study on alcohol education and young people[3] compared a peer-led programme to a teacher-led programme and to no programme at all in 25 schools in Australia, Chile, Norway and Swaziland. The educational programme emphasized refusal skills for alcohol use among eighth and ninth graders in the four countries. The peer-led educational programme appeared to be efficacious in reducing adolescent involvement with alcohol across a variety of settings, economies and cultures. The study confirmed that peer leaders are unique in their ability to influence peer group behaviour because they are themselves members of the peer group; as such, they offer credible role models and as they utilize the same language as their peers, they prove to be very effective disseminators of social information. It was found that peer leaders can be trained to modify environmental, personality and behavioural factors that are predictive of alcohol use among adolescents, and become a viable alternative to teachers and adult leaders.

The child-to-child approach[4] is no less exciting. Throughout the developing world, many children spend much of their lives looking after younger sisters and brothers. Why not teach these child-minders simple facts about health and help them do a better job of caring for their younger siblings? This question brought David Morley, under the umbrella of the University of London, to involve teaching experts from many parts of the world in developing very practical teaching materials called "activity sheets". The object is to involve children, beyond the school, in activities at home and in the community.

The philosophy of the child-to-child or youth-to-youth approach is founded on the belief that positive peer influence and social support are powerful and effective means of promoting lifestyles conducive to health. Its success shows that different generations working together as well as mixing of professional and lay groups can lead to comprehensive programmes that really work.

The Work Site

Moving on to the adult world and more specifically to the workplace, we find some very good programmes which tackle occupational health and safety from a broad perspective covering legislative policy, corporate cultural change and the quality of working life. Many such programmes show positive results whether they deal with high blood pressure, smoking cessation, cholesterol and weight reduction or fitness.

What is behind their success? Three factors stand out:

- First, these programmes recognise the dynamic interdependence of the worker and his work within an ecological framework: they avoid focussing on an individual risk factor approach.
- Second, they provide opportunities for the work group itself to change the environment, to redesign the physical work space, to improve the food in cafeterias and to make suggestions for work organisation.

- Last, but not least, the programmes benefit from the joint support of management, employers and the unions.

According to Weinstein[5], no programme can ever succeed in the long run without such support and experience shows it is essential to establish contacts at top levels with senior union leaders.

Health insurance companies are another partner of health promotion on the worksite. In many countries, especially in the United States, they are becoming a major force in the promotion of lifestyles conducive to health as they are keen on diminishing the cost of sickness claims.

As regards the HIV-infected person, exclusion from the workplace remains a serious problem with its negative impact on self-esteem, the threat to financial stability and the loss of significant social relationships. Appropriate public health and social policies are urgently needed, together with suitable health rules and regulations to ensure that the right to work of HIV-infected persons is respected and to facilitate their integration in the working community.

Maternal and Child Health

Maternal and child health and family planning programmes are in a very special position when it comes to stopping the spread of AIDS. There is no doubt that their staff represent the largest pool of health personnel most able to help in the control of AIDS. They have long experience in counselling and dealing with the many aspects of sexuality that are all related to the prevention of HIV transmission.

I would like to use this setting to draw attention to an aspect of planning that we tend to minimise in evolving health promotion programmes. It deals with practical aspects which show vividly the interdependence of health work with other sectors. I am thinking of developing country situations where factors totally beyond the scope of the health services influence the availability of such essential supplies as condoms or plastic aprons, soap, gloves. These factors include slow transport, slow communication, space for storage, inadequate central planning or budgeting.

The best education programme will fall flat if logistic support fails. Good advice is of little value when means to implement it are not available. In fact, health promotion goes much further. It simply says, *"Make healthy choices the easy choices"*.

Health foods are a case in point. Recently, nutrition programmes[6] showed clearly that three problems must be tackled simultaneously: providing adequate information; making the foods easily accessible; and making them available at a competitive price.

If we turn to the problem of HIV transmission through the sharing of drug injection equipment, it has become increasingly clear that exhortations not to do so need to be supported by easy access to clean injecting equipment. However, this implies acknowledgment at policy level that the spread of HIV is a greater threat to individual and public health than drug misuse.

STD Services: An Entry Point

Coordination between AIDS and STD programmes stands as a most natural step. In fact, the extent of coordination varies from country to country and is often related to the strength of the country's STD programme at the time when AIDS first appeared. Interactions range from the peripheral level, where information can be shared through joint planning and implementation, to the central level from which both programmes are sometimes run by a single manager.

The growing interest in close coordination between AIDS and STD programmes[7] is easily understood as many of the measures for preventing sexual transmission of HIV and STDs are similar and target audiences for these interventions are practically the same. STD clinical services represent an important access point for persons at high risk of AIDS since there is a strong association between the occurrence of HIV infection and the presence of STDs. Mutual learning, here, seems more synonymous with coordination and *structural* measures to minimise duplication of staff and increase overall programme effectiveness.

But more is needed. As Don Nutbeam[8] stresses, clinical services must be made more accessible, approachable, and generally "consumer friendly", especially for marginalised groups. He cites stimulating examples from countries such as The Netherlands, where STD services have been developed as part of substantial outreach programmes directed at workers in the sex industry. Here, access to disease screening and counselling is included in programmes which offer practical and pragmatic support as well, including condoms and facilities for rest and showers.

Moulding service provisions around consumer needs and reorienting health services to make them fully relevant and accessible to vulnerable and marginalised groups remains a major challenge for the 1990s.

At Community Level: Some Exciting Perspectives

These perspectives include the Healthy Cities project with which you are certainly familiar. This project was initiated five years ago by WHO/EURO and its rapid development clearly reflects growing awareness of the need for health promotion to develop methods and mechanisms that support integrative strategies[9].

As the Vienna Dialogue IV pointed out:

> "The development of infrastructures is a strategic process. Each country or situation will vary over time, therefore there is a need to take advantage of all opportunities in the system to develop health promotion. It is vital to be aware of the entry points and one should capitalise on opportunities in one's environment in order to cope with the many barriers and constraints."[10]

This statement could serve to define the very objective of the National AIDS Committees which represent a key mechanism to develop AIDS programmes and to promote linkages with other sectors and mutual learning. Such structures exist today in some 160 countries and bring together expertise from many different fields in planning strategies.

Some have proved very effective in supporting an integrative approach, others less, but all serve to implement an essential process of health promotion by setting the stage for dynamic interaction between people from all walks of life: medical specialists, lay persons, decision makers, people with AIDS, religious leaders, and many others. The development of these committees, worldwide, exemplifies the use of a simple infrastructure to promote horizontal processes which facilitate linkages between sectors at the community level.

Coping with the Stress of Illness

At this point I would like to reflect with you on an aspect of the health promotion concept which has special relevance for persons who are infected with HIV or have AIDS. At the heart of health promotion, we find the notion of the health *potential* that exists in each individual. For Kickbusch[11] this health potential means that *"there are aspects of health and well being that can, or could, develop from whatever point one starts in life, whether as a wonderfully healthy baby or as somebody who has already gone through a lot of life crises"*. In other words, health promotion is concerned with enabling people *"to maximise their health potential and move ahead"*.

The field of chronic illness provides us with many examples indicating that people can develop a new quality of health and life despite serious illness. According to Milz[12], adapting successfully to chronic illness means *"finding a way of life that sustains hope, diminishes fear, and preserves a quality of living that takes account of the limitations associated with the illness"*. This adaptation requires the development of new relationships on a variety of levels. This leads us to the need for enhancing people's capacity to cope with chronic conditions.

Lazarus[13] indicates that the capacity to cope better with the stresses of illness, or help others to do so, depends on the appraisal, by the individual concerned, of the source of harm and its threat to his or her well being. The patient with chronic illness is continually appraising symptoms, pains, and disease progression with respect to their significance for his survival and tries to cope accordingly.

In this process of coping, social support stands out as a most important factor in reducing the level of stress and enabling people to regain a sense of coherence, to keep a self-concept that is realistic and positive. Sources of social support are found in social networks, inter-personal processes, and religion, as well as in the socially defined roles which structure our daily activities.

Lerner[14] reports on what he calls "a social phenomenon" among cancer patients who have chosen to engage actively in the fight for recovery and are searching for personal strategies of intensive health promotion. Today, there are literally hundreds of self help groups, support organisations and health centres for cancer patients in countries around the world. They are developing innovative programmes for coming to terms with the manifold problems triggered off by diagnosis of the illness and its treatment. The focus is often on creating an environment in which people with cancer can be helped professionally and can help each other. These experiences provide a growing body of evidence that a great deal can be done to enhance well-being through improved coping skills and reinforced social support.

This should not detract from the fact that some factors lie beyond the ability of the individual to influence his or her well-being. Consider the quality of foodstuffs, their composition and processing, and their availability: some chronic pain conditions like migraine or rheumatic pain may be indications of foodstuff or chemical environmental incompatibilities. Such observations further reinforce the need for health promotion to involve many sectors in finding solutions.

To conclude, this brief overview leaves us with two important messages:

First, at the level of health planning:

- The promotion of health cannot be achieved by the health sector alone. Health promotion demands coordinated action by all concerned. It means shaping health public policy that aims to combine complementary approaches including legislation, fiscal measures and organisational changes. It means creating supportive environments and strengthening community action.

The second message concerns the individual:

- At the heart of health promotion is the notion of the health potential that exists in each person and can be developed at whatever stage of health in life.

    Let me share with you a moving statement from a person who is coping successfully with AIDS for ten years now — yes, ten years:

    > *"We are the ones living on the frontline and we can offer an expertise that cannot be learnt elsewhere. We are men and women with knowledge and skills, talents and abilities, hopes and dreams and, indeed, health. We are the ones who can exemplify the importance of the human ideal of solidarity instilled in this epidemic to the world."*[15]

    Mutual understanding ... Building links ... Beyond planning and practical problems, this objective illuminates the inner motivation of health action: I mean, solidarity.

References

1. World Health Organisation. Ottawa Charter for Health Promotion. Copenhagen/Geneva: WHO, 1986.

2. Hastings G. Young people, sex and social marketing. Paper presented at Family Planning Association National Conference on "Promoting Sexual Health and Family Planning", London 22 November 1990.

3. World Health Organisation. The health of youth. Technical discussion paper A 42/2. Geneva: WHO, 1989.

4. Webb J. From child to child. Geneva: WHO/SCIPHE, Education for Health 1985; **No 2**: 27-30.

5. Weinstein M. Experiences of Success. *In:* Federal Centre for Health Education in Collaboration with WHO. Health promotion in the working world. Heidelberg/New York: Springer, 1989.

6. Holm L-E. Nutritional intervention studies in cancer prevention. Med Oncol & Tumor Pharmacother 1990; **7**: 209-215.

7. World Health Organisation. Consensus statement from the Consultation on Global Strategies for Coordination of AIDS and STD Control Programmes, Geneva 11-13 July 1990. WHO/GPA/INF/90.2. Geneva: WHO, 1990. *Unpublished document.*

8. Nutbeam D. Health Promotion and the AIDS epidemic. Paper presented at the European Workshop on Social and Cultural Issues in HIV Prevention through Health Promotion. Brussels, 18-20 January 1990.

9. World Health Organisation. Healthy Cities Project: a project becomes a movement. Review of Progress 1987 to 1990. Copenhagen: WHO, 1990.

10. World Health Organisation. Vienna Dialogue IV: Pioneering health promotion: Structures for new public health. Copenhagen: WHO, 1989.

11. Kickbusch I. Enhancing people's health potential. *In:* Kaplun A (ed). Health promotion and chronic illness: Discovering a new quality of life. (WHO Regional Publications, European series, No. 44). Copenhagen: WHO, 1991.

12. Milz H. Healthy ill persons - social cynicism or new perspectives for living with a chronic illness. *In:* Kaplun A (ed). Health promotion and chronic illness: Discovering a new quality of life. (WHO Regional Publications, European series, No. 44). Copenhagen: WHO, 1991.

13. Lazarus R. Coping with the stresses of Illness. *In:* Kaplun A (ed). Health promotion and chronic illness: Discovering a new quality of life. (WHO Regional Publications, European series, No. 44). Copenhagen: WHO, 1991.

14. Lerner M. Emerging forces in cancer care. *In:* Kaplun A (ed). Health promotion and chronic illness: Discovering a new quality of life. (WHO Regional Publications, European series, No. 44). Copenhagen: WHO, 1991.

15. Rector R. Maximising the existing health potential of people with HIV/AIDS: Have we succeeded? Geneva: WHO, AIDS Health Promotion Exchange 1991; **No 1**.

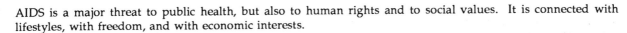

7

HIV/AIDS: Ethical and Legal Perspectives — the European Context

Henriette Roscam Abbing
University of Limburg and
Dutch Ministry of Health, Welfare and Cultural Affairs

Introduction

The particularities of HIV transmission are well known. It is spread primarily through sexual contact. Unlike most other sexually transmittable diseases, AIDS is lethal. In the absence of a vaccine or cure for HIV infection, prevention is the only method of avoiding the devastating effects of the disease.

AIDS is a major threat to public health, but also to human rights and to social values. It is connected with lifestyles, with freedom, and with economic interests.

Strategies designed to prevent the sexual transmission of diseases should in general take into account various ethical and legal aspects involved. In particular in the event of HIV, a balance should be found between the interests of the individual, his or her autonomy and privacy on the one hand, and the interests of society in being protected against health risks on the other hand. But there is more to it. In the fight against AIDS, the protection of health also brings about a need to balance various distinct individual human rights.

To be effective, programmes to prevent HIV infection through sexual contact should be constructed in such a manner that discrimination is avoided and that the free and full access to societal attainments is secured. Any preventive scheme which does not take these requisites into account is counterproductive.

It must be recognised that AIDS, because of its special characteristics, entails more complicated legal issues than other STDs. There is, for instance, a latency period prior to discovering the infection; symptoms appear long after a person has become contagious, and so forth. Moreover, as mentioned earlier, AIDS remains a fatal disease, despite recent advances with treatment methods.

At present some medicaments postpone the development of AIDS related symptoms, but no more. The disease still remains lethal; the medicaments do not change the contagiousness nor the methods of transmission. Hence, the legal issues also remain. And yet, the prospects of medication and the increasing possibilities of early intervention are likely to create expectations which are not justified; they can also negatively influence the prevention message of policies for promoting sexual health. There is, therefore, all the more reason not to relax the human rights aspects in this framework.

Human Rights and the Public Health Rationale

The observance of the human rights and dignity of individuals in all areas of health follows from the principle of autonomy and the right to self-determination. These principles lie at the basis of various human rights instruments, including the UN Covenant on Civil and Political Rights (1966) and the European Convention on Human Rights and Fundamental Freedoms (Council of Europe, 1948). These principles find expression in, for instance, the right to equal treatment and the right to privacy, which also covers the right to bodily integrity. The reason for the particular concern to protect human rights and dignity in the fight against AIDS is that there is a strong public health rationale. Human rights must be respected because they are inherent in people as human beings[1]. In the case of AIDS, this is not only a moral imperative and a legal requirement. It is also critical to the success of national and international health promotion programmes. Discrimination, stigmatisation and exclusion from society of HIV infected persons does not help them to assume responsibility for preventing HIV transmission to others; it is unjustified in public health terms and may, conversely, endanger public health. Therefore, the protection of the rights and dignity of HIV infected persons has become an integral part of the Global Strategy on AIDS of WHO[2] and of other international organisations, such as the Council of Europe and the European Communities. These organisations emphasise the importance of anti-discrimination and anti-stigmatisation efforts. Only when measures to limit the spread of HIV comply with the principles embedded in international human rights instruments, can the personal and social impact of HIV infection be reduced.

Public health is formally allowed as one of the exceptions which may give grounds for restricting human rights. It is, however, a rare exception and, if applied at all, it must not lead to infringement of the non-discrimination principle. However, to use public health as a pretext to limit human rights in the case of HIV infection and AIDS is, in general, not based on a public health rationale and is likely to be counterproductive to preventive undertakings.

Education, Information and Counselling and Human Rights

To date, education, information and counselling on how to avoid exposure to, or transmission of, HIV infection are the only useful methods to prevent the spread of the disease.

Sexual health programmes can be developed at three levels: the population at large, at schoolchildren, at special target groups which are at risk through their behaviour (prostitutes, IV drug users) or through other reasons (prisoners, health care providers), or can take place in an individual setting, such as at STD clinics. Each scheme creates its own set of ethical and legal issues in relation to human rights and dignity. Various factors can hamper the educational outreach of programmes specifically designed to prevent HIV infection through sexual transmission. These factors include the spiritual and cultural characteristics of a country, the extent of stigmatisation and discrimination as a result of HIV infection or suspicion of HIV infection, and the impact of HIV infection on the availability of necessary social services, such as employment, housing, insurance and the like. Some of the topical issues are discussed in the following sections.

Religious Convictions, Human Rights, and the Public Health Rationale

The AIDS epidemic may well necessitate reconsideration of some of the practical consequences of religious and/or culturally determined policies. There is, for instance, the evident question of how to accommodate religious freedom with the need to protect society from serious diseases.

The limitation or prohibition of, for instance, sexual education as part of health education at schools, or of the free sale of condoms, is unnecessary from the point of view of the right to freedom of religion. It is, moreover, counterproductive to the prevention of the sexual transmission of diseases.

In fact, there is a strong public health argument in favour of health education, including sexual health education. The right to freedom of thought, conscience and religion is an individual human right, to be protected by governments. But this does not imply that policies which are based solely on religious or moral convictions can be imposed on others who hold different views. Pluriformity of society has to be accepted. Such restrictive policies are contrary to individual freedom. Governments that restrict sexual education at schools or the availability of condoms, solely on religious or moral grounds, act against the fundaments of individual human rights and against their meaning. They are also likely to come into conflict with the right to education and the right to freely acquire information. Freedom of religion does not equate with the imposition of religious convictions by governmental measures. This is the more serious when the imposition of religious convictions poses a serious threat to the health of people, as might well be the case with HIV/AIDS. Religious convictions, if dealt with in this way, can seriously hamper the public health programme to prevent HIV infection, because education and information are its cornerstones.

Instead, in case of sexual transmission of diseases and in particular HIV infection, the protection of public health is a cause for government to promote, and not to restrict, health education and sexual education as part of it. If necessary, public health can even be a formally accepted ground to restrict the freedom of religion. In accordance with for instance the European Human Rights Convention's jurisprudence, this can be the case if such a restriction meets with the condition of necessity in a democratic society for the protection of a legitimate aim; that is, there is a pressing social need, there is no less intrusive alternative, the restriction is effective and proportional to that need, weighed both against its adverse effects on the persons on whom it is imposed and against the public interest in the free exercise of the right concerned. To give just one example, in curative medical care it is generally accepted that parental authority may not be used against the health interest of a minor. Parental choices may thus be overruled if they entail a serious threat to the minor. There is no justification not to apply this rule similarly to promotion of sexual health, whether or not it takes the form of education.

Testing and Human Rights

Another issue in preventing sexual transmission of HIV is testing. Testing is a useful instrument in health care when deployed as a detection instrument for treatable STDs. Its legitimacy as part of an HIV prevention programme should be scrutinised very carefully against the possible implications for the individual (and his or her partner). Because of the problems involved, HIV testing and screening may be intrusive and cost-ineffective, diverting scarce resources from education programmes.

Despite advances in treatment methods, in particular the possibilities for early intervention in an asymptomatic phase, there is at present no justification to replace the present restrictive approach to testing and screening policies by a promotional one. In the present state of the art, to implement obligatory testing within sexual health promotion policies will pose serious problems in respect of free, informed consent, privacy, stigmatisation and discrimination and will have social consequences (in terms of employment and insurance); it is likely to hinder the outreach of the preventive message. One of the first conditions to be met when HIV testing is considered, is to ensure free consent, on the basis of full, objective information. This applies not only to the prospects of the disease, but also to the possible consequences of a positive outcome, to measures taken to avoid these consequences and the like.

Compulsory testing of certain groups particularly at risk, such as prostitutes, is difficult to carry out. It will certainly not contribute to successful prevention, because it will drive them underground. Compulsory testing has produced a low yield; it is counterproductive and, moreover, unnecessary because of the methods of transmission. Education and information should instead be specially focussed on target groups of this kind.

Negative effects of testing, in the framework of programmes for promoting sexual health with a view to prevent HIV infection, include avoidance of detection and contact with health and social services and "driving underground" of those who have an increased risk of exposure to HIV, hence putting them out of reach of information and education. It is of paramount importance to recognise and understand in time the legal complications and human rights issues involved with testing. HIV testing cannot contribute to prevention if confidentiality is not ensured; if confidential counselling and other support services to HIV infected people and people with AIDS are unavailable, insufficient or lacking; if seropositivity or AIDS is a notifiable named disease; or if test results are disclosed to third parties without the consent of the person concerned. If policies and programmes for promoting sexual health do not take into account these issues, then testing is a threat to the privacy of the person concerned, with serious consequences for his or her possibilities of social functioning.

Only when voluntary, anonymous and unlinked testing is available, without any pressure to undergo testing, together with information, education and counselling services to encourage abandonment of high-risk behaviour, may HIV transmission be prevented.

Yet another issue is contact-tracing. In the case of sexually transmittable diseases, privacy and medical secrecy always pose problems because of conflicting interests, whereas part of STD control is contact-tracing and partner notification. Questions then arise about the extent of the medical secrecy, about the duty to warn versus the right not to be informed and the like. In case of HIV in particular, there is cause of concern when contact-tracing and partner notification are urged. A requisite for any such policy is the free participation and consent of the individual who has tested positively. If the infected individual refuses to inform his or her partner, or refuses to allow his or her partner to be informed by the health care provider, there is a real dilemma. Health care providers and counsellors then face a conflict of duties. The advantages and disadvantages of informing the partner have to be weighed against each other in the individual circumstances. This is all the more so in the case of HIV, because of its lethality. The partner is not free to refuse the information; he or she will be uncertain whether or not he or she is infected, which is inhuman, and in fact contrary to an individual's right not to be informed; pressure to undergo testing is almost unavoidable, which in turn is contrary to the requisite of free and informed consent. Routinely informing the partner against the wishes of the infected individual in addition creates a problem of breach of medical secrecy, thus undermining confidence in STD services and health care workers in general. Therefore, prior to carrying out the HIV test, consideration should be given to how to deal with seropositivity in relation to a partner. It should be clear from the outset that information will be given to a partner against the wishes of the HIV infected person only in the case of a serious risk of transmission (for instance pregnancy). If there are doubts about medical secrecy, individuals likely to be infected will avoid using the services of STD clinics, thus adding to the risk of transmission. Indeed, the breach of medical secrecy in a situation of a conflict of duties is generally acceptable only in exceptional circumstances, where certain conditions are met:

- the utmost effort has been made to obtain consent;
- the health care provider faces serious compunctions of conscience;
- there is no other way to solve the problem;
- not to breach secrecy could cause serious harm to a third party;
- there is reasonable certainty that the harm will be prevented by the breach of secrecy.

HIV Testing and Social Consequences

Preventing of transmission of HIV may also be hindered because of societal consequences of HIV testing, even if anonymity is respected. As long as employers or insurance companies, for instance, are free to make use of and discriminate on the basis of information on HIV testing, whether or not this is limited to the mere fact of the test having been carried out (eg in unlinked anonymous seroprevalence studies), individuals who have reason to suspect infection will evade testing and thus miss education and counselling. They will then be beyond the reach of advice to abandon high-risk behaviour in order to avoid HIV transmission. HIV screening and testing involves the collection of highly sensitive medical information. Disclosure of such information to third parties without the person's consent, or under pressure, in order to attain socially necessary services, infringes upon a person's right to privacy and jeopardises his or her possibilities for living as an integrated part of society. The social consequences of HIV testing can be serious. They may include isolation, economic loss, restrictions of opportunities for insurance, employment, schooling, housing and the like[3].

Moreover, caution is needed, now in particular, because the possibilities of early intervention are likely to encourage people who have reason to suspect HIV infection to undergo testing. To balance the relative benefits of early intervention for the individual and the social consequences, which can be destructive, special urgency must now attend the issues of free, fully informed consent and confidentiality.

The Role of the Legislator

Because HIV is transmitted by sexual contacts, it is closely linked to the intimate human sphere and to privacy. Intrusions upon the individual sphere require strong arguments and necessitate a clear legislative basis. As was seen before, public health may constitute an argument for restrictive legislation. Such measures must however be justified in terms of effectiveness and proportionality.

To prevent HIV infection effectively, the legislator can certainly play a role. In the case of AIDS, invasions of privacy and restrictions on individual liberty, imposed by the law to protect public safety, will not result in a clear public health benefit; they will not contribute to prevention, and will ultimately compromise the democratic fabric of society. Instead, public health measures adopted by governments which promote education and information on sexual health, as well as counselling, while fully respecting individual human rights and dignity, will yield better results in preventing the spread of AIDS.

A wise legislator steers clear of measures which restrict individual human rights and liberties, because in case of HIV/AIDS, there is no public health rationale to do so.

A wise legislator protects individuals in society, prevents discrimination and stigmatisation, and ensures equal treatment and equal possibilities for participation in social attainments, so that education and information reaches those who have to be reached and that serological testing as part of programmes to prevent the sexual transmission of HIV will become as acceptable as diagnosing any other STD.

AIDS is an infectious disease and should not be considered as a separate category in the frame of policies to promote sexual health. It should not be dealt with in an isolated legislative approach either[4].

AIDS is a test-case of how seriously society takes equal protection and equal possibilities for every citizen. Only when health education and health promotion are based on a social approach and fully respect human rights and dignity, is the prevention of the spread of HIV through sexual transmission likely to be effective.

References

1. UN Centre for Human Rights, WHO. AIDS and human rights, Final document, HR/AIDS/1989/3, 10. Geneva: UNCHR, 1990.

2. Mann J M. AIDS, discrimination and public health. Geneva: WHO, 1988, 1.

3. WHO. Report of the meeting on criteria for HIV screening programmes. WHO/SPA/87.2. Geneva: WHO, 1987, 8.

4. WHO Regional Office for Europe. Health legislation and ethics in the field of AIDS and HIV infection. Copenhagen: WHO, 1988, 17.

8

New Directions for Health Promotion
to Prevent HIV Infection and other STDs

William W Darrow and Ronald O Valdiserri
Centers for Disease Control
Atlanta

(Oral presentation by Dr Darrow)

We begin by reviewing the first 10 years of the HIV/AIDS epidemic, the research and policy issues addressed during our first decade with HIV/AIDS, and the objectives of public information programmes created to let people know about HIV/AIDS. Then we present five directions that we believe health education and health promotion programmes should take to reduce the incidence of HIV infection. After we outline each proposal, we attempt to illustrate and illuminate each suggestion. We conclude that more must be done to personalise the impact of the epidemic if we are to achieve more universal support for HIV/AIDS prevention and the promotion of sexual health.

Review: the First Decade of the HIV/AIDS Epidemic

In London, on January 26, 1988, Jonathan Mann[1], past director of the World Health Organisation's Global Programme on AIDS, reviewed the three stages of the HIV/AIDS epidemic at the World Summit of Ministers of Health on Programmes for AIDS Prevention. In the 1970s, human immunodeficiency virus (HIV) spread silently and extensively among persons who engaged in certain behaviours in certain parts of the world. AIDS was first recognised in Spring 1981 and steps were taken immediately after that to define the extent of this public health problem in the United States and some other countries. Although some community-based organisations, such as the Kaposi's Sarcoma Foundation of San Francisco and the Gay Men's Health Crisis of New York City, were formed in the early 1980s to provide risk-reduction information and services, many governments did not mobilise to confront the full threat of the HIV/AIDS epidemic until the mid-1980s, or later.

The detection of AIDS in 1981 led to a series of research and public policy issues. First, scientists set out to find the cause of AIDS through sequential epidemiological and laboratory investigations and to describe HIV transmission patterns through case, case-control, and cohort studies. Once an acceptable case definition was developed, the prevalence of AIDS could be estimated in various populations and, after a reliable antibody test was developed and approved in 1985, HIV prevalence and incidence trends could be assessed. As knowledge about transmission patterns and the possibility of a blood-borne agent emerged, public health guidelines and policies were formulated and implemented to prevent sexual, perinatal, and needle or syringe-sharing transmissions, and to protect blood supplies.

As early as 1983, the San Francisco Health Department responded to early reports of AIDS and preliminary epidemiological findings from a case-control study of AIDS in homosexual and bisexual men by preparing and disseminating a poster (figure 1). However, national campaigns such as "America Responds to AIDS", designed to alert the public to the cause and extent of the HIV/AIDS problem, were not introduced until several years later.

Public information campaigns introduced in 1986 or later generally had three objectives:

1.   To inform everyone about the cause of AIDS and the established routes of HIV transmission;

2.   To reduce anxieties about infection with HIV through sharing eating utensils or other types of casual contact with infected persons; and

3.   To build popular support for effective and efficient programmes to prevent further transmission of HIV and to assist persons infected with HIV.

Public opinion surveys and other measures of knowledge and belief, such as the AIDS Supplement to the Health Interview Survey conducted in the United States by the National Center for Health Statistics[2,3], suggest that these three objectives were accomplished in the 1980s.

HIV/AIDS in the 1990s

We propose five major directions for health education and the promotion of sexual health in the 1990s:

1.   Targetted messages for persons who remain at risk of acquiring or transmitting HIV infection that require their involvement and are based on appraisals of their current state with respect to stages of behavioural change;

2.   Assessment of the effectiveness of interventions designed to change behaviours, based upon the abilities of the intervention to move persons with high-risk behaviours to lower- or no-risk behaviours in incremental stages;

3.   Analysis of the social and cultural contexts in which interventions are developed, applied and evaluated;

4.   Integration of HIV/AIDS prevention efforts with STD prevention, drug misuse prevention, and family planning efforts so that persons at risk for adverse social outcomes are better able to make decisions that lead to healthier consequences;

5.   Evaluation of the extent to which planned interventions and other activities contribute to the overall goal of sexual health.

Targetted messages

Some health education and promotion programmes were developed in the 1980s with representatives of target groups involved as consultants, focus-group members, or key informants; in many cases community-based and national minority organisations took the lead in developing and implementing health education/risk reduction messages and other intervention activities. Our first proposal recommends that these activities continue and expand to include persons at risk working with technical specialists in the iterative processes of assessment, intervention and evaluation. We are calling for greater communication and collaboration between social scientists, for example, with their conceptual schemes suggesting that persons at risk for HIV and other adverse outcomes usually move through a series of steps before they change their behaviour[4], and those persons who are struggling to accept new information about themselves and are attempting to modify their behaviours based on this information.

For example, the California Prostitutes Education Project (Cal-PEP) developed a manual for identifying and contacting women in the sex industry and recruiting them to safer sex workshops by offering door prizes[5]. During the workshops, various methods of HIV/STD prevention were described and discussed. Participants were given opportunities to develop technical as well as interpersonal skills. We believe that some of these workshops were evaluated in terms of information transfer, but we have not seen the results of systematic attempts to evaluate their effectiveness in terms of impact (eg increased usage of condoms during vaginal intercourse by workshop participants) or outcome (eg reduced incidence of gonorrhoea). This example is offered to suggest how researchers might help evaluate the messages targetted for, and experiences of, sex industry women in San Francisco and elsewhere.

Other examples include poster slogans: "AIDS is scary, but a zit is real. Right?" stressing that AIDS is something that a young man should talk about; that a condom can be a "Life preserver"; it "Stops transmission fluid leaks"; it is "Smart sportswear for the active man"; and that he will be "No less a man for playing safe". These messages, developed and implemented by or with persons at risk, appear to have been created with the knowledge that behaviour changes are accomplished through a series of stages, that each step is usually carefully taken, and such steps must be continually reinforced to maintain behaviour change.

Assessment of interventions

Roy M Anderson and Robert M May[6] have used mathematical models to explain HIV transmission dynamics in human populations. A key element in predicting the future course of the epidemic is the "reproductive rate" (R_o). The reproductive rate is determined by the product of the number of new partners exposed through unprotected sexual intercourse by a person infected with HIV, the transmission probability per exposure, and the duration of infectiousness. When R_o exceeds unity, the epidemic expands. When R_o is less than unity, the epidemic contracts. Therefore a major goal of health education and promotion in the 1990s should be to reduce the reproductive rate to less than 1.0.

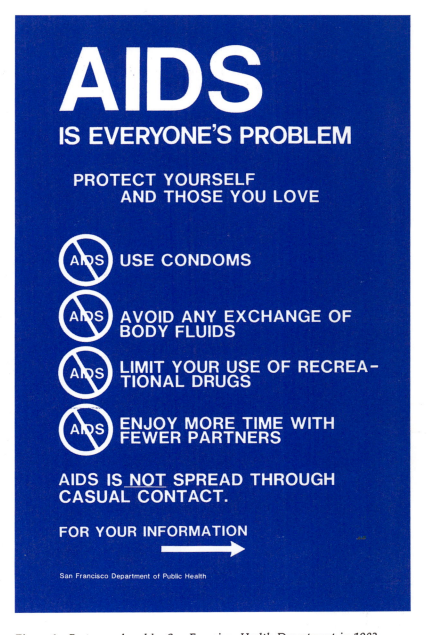

Figure 1: *Poster produced by San Francisco Health Department in 1983.*

The content of interventions will vary depending on many factors, including the prevalence of HIV infection in the population of interest, the characteristics of the target group, and the behavioural objective(s) of the intervention; but the goal might include one or more of the three components contained in the Anderson-May model: 1) reduce the number of new sexual (or needle or syringe-sharing) partners acquired per unit of time; 2) reduce the number of unprotected sexual exposures; and/or 3) reduce the period of time in which the infected person is infectious. To assess the effectiveness of the intervention, we must measure the extent to which the intervention is delivered to and received by the target group (process evaluation) as well as the extent to which the behavioural objective is attained (impact evaluation) and the incidence of infection is reduced (outcome evaluation). A crucial point is that we should not necessarily be disappointed if our interventions often fall short of our behavioural objectives, but we should accept responsibility if we cannot adequately describe and explain our shortcomings.

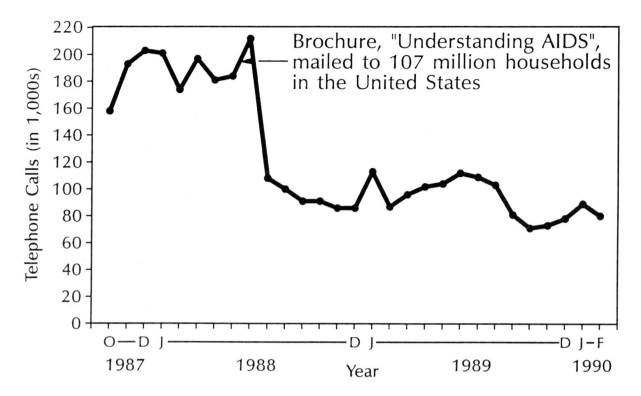

Figure 2: Calls to the US National AIDS Hotline, 1987-90.

For instance, in several Western countries, government officials developed brochures, copies of which were mailed to every household or postal address. The brochure sent to every postal patron in the United States provided facts about the cause of AIDS and transmission patterns of the "AIDS virus"; attempted to dispel myths; and encouraged persons who wanted more specific information about prevention to call a toll-free, national telephone hotline. Data from public opinion polls and the AIDS Supplement to the Health Interview Survey showed that the mail-out helped increase awareness and correct some misunderstandings among persons who received and read the brochure. Telephone calls to the national hotline peaked shortly after the mail-out and then decreased rapidly (figure 2).

By many measures the national mail-out was successful in blanketing the nation with standardised information about AIDS, and in motivating selected persons to call for specific, personalised information about HIV/AIDS prevention. However, the mail-out to 107 million residences and postal addresses in the United States failed to reach housing quarters without mailboxes. Many men and women who inject drugs and engage in other high risk behaviours are homeless or reside in settings where they cannot be reached by mail.

For injecting drug users not enrolled in treatment programmes, outreach programmes have been designed, developed and implemented to contact persons at risk for HIV/AIDS and to refer them to clinical facilities where they can be tested for HIV antibodies and offered other services. The number of persons tested for HIV antibodies and the number who have tested positive have increased since anonymous or confidential testing was first offered in public sites in 1985, but now many facilities in the US are crowded and overwhelmed with the demand for services. The problem is acute in many state and local health departments where services have been reduced or eliminated. For example, in Sacramento County, California, local officials were invited to replicate a study of 2,358 STD clinic patients which CDC and local officials had conducted 20 years earlier in Summer 1971 in a centrally located, walk-in, well-staffed and well-equipped clinic. Because of budget cuts brought on by a tax reform movement in 1978, Sacramento County could no longer support an STD clinic; persons with genitourinary complaints now must go to private providers, hospital emergency rooms, primary care clinics or elsewhere for the diagnosis and treatment of STDs. In many societies, including the United States, the public health

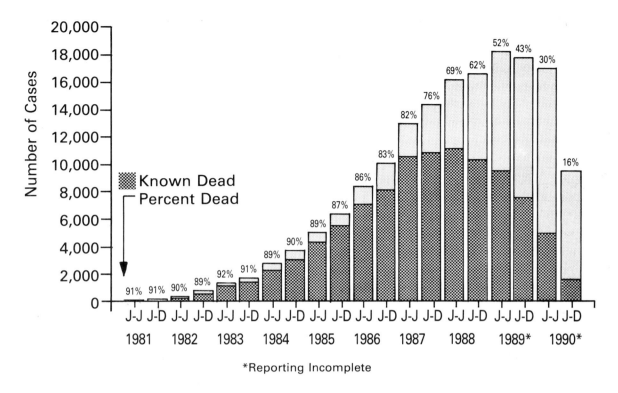

Figure 3: Cases of AIDS and case-fatality rates by half-year of diagnosis, reported 1981 through 1990, United States.

infrastructure cannot provide and deliver basic services, such as adequate risk-reduction counselling, free testing for HIV and other STDs, confidential post-test counselling and provider-assisted partner notification.

Understanding context

The HIV/AIDS epidemic has now been with us long enough to have a past. Those of us who met and worked with persons who were among the first to be diagnosed with AIDS can remember the feelings they expressed: anger about what had happened to them; denial that AIDS was threatening their lives, the lives of their loved ones, and their lifestyles; acceptance of their illness and its impact on social life; and then affirmation of the dignity and sanctity of life. Similarly, enough time has passed and enough studies have been reported for us to realise that the social processes stimulated by the HIV/AIDS epidemic have been similar in many different parts of the world. The social patterns we have witnessed with HIV/AIDS are remarkably similar to those described in historical accounts of syphilis[7,8,9] and responses to Legionnaires' disease in more recent history[10]. Although there have been unique aspects to various epidemics described in historical records, and to the reactions to HIV/AIDS observed in different cultures, comparative analyses suggest that when we understand their context, we can continue to learn from one another in the 1990s through our common experiences with HIV disease, STDs and other socio-medical problems, such as drug misuse, pregnancy planning, and efforts to control other infectious diseases.

Integration of activities

Because available resources are limited and there is some evidence that prevention programmes and clinical services require greater coordination, we recommend that attempts to integrate activities in a more comprehensive (as opposed to categorical) approach be initiated or, in many cases, continued. The overall goal of this proposal is to promote more responsible health decision-making in general. However, in making this broad proposal, we recognise that the behavioural objectives and expected outcomes of specific interventions may differ.

Rate (per 100,000 population)

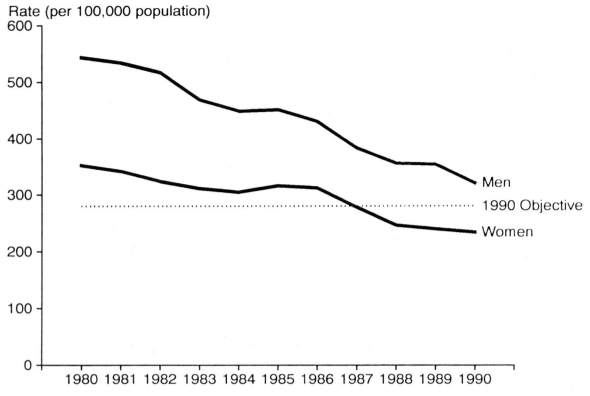

Source: CDC.

Figure 4: Gonorrhoea: rates by gender, United States, 1980-90, and 1990 goal.

For example, in the United States, the number of cases of AIDS reported over six-month intervals increased steadily from 1981 to 1987 and then began to level off in 1988 (figure 3). During the 1980s, reported rates of gonorrhoea steadily declined to the target objective set by the Public Health Service for 1990 (figure 4). These data might suggest that HIV/AIDS prevention efforts were spilling over to prevent another, more common, sexually transmitted disease: gonorrhoea. However, primary and secondary syphilis cases reported in the United States declined from 1982 to 1986, especially among men, and then began to rise in the midst of an aggressive campaign to prevent HIV/AIDS (figure 5). The number of reported cases of congenital syphilis in the United States is now significantly higher than it was during the decade before AIDS was detected (figure 6). These three sexually transmitted infections — HIV, gonorrhoea, and syphilis — could be circulating in different networks of the sexually active population, or perhaps, are responding to different influences in similar networks or groups.

Surveys of never-married men aged 17, 18 and 19 in 1979[11] and again in 1988[12] in the United States suggest that the proportion who reported ever engaging in sexual intercourse increased (table 1), but the proportion who reported using a condom during their last episode of sexual intercourse increased to a greater extent (table 2). Even more recently published findings from the National Survey of Family Growth, Cycle IV[13], confirm these results among a representative sample of women 15-19 years old living in households in the United States, suggesting that health promotion programmes are facilitating more frequent condom use, but are not deterring young people from engaging in sexual intercourse. Thus, the proportion of young persons susceptible to HIV and other STDs has expanded since early reports of AIDS, but the behaviour of the sexually active population has changed in response to messages about safer sexual practices.

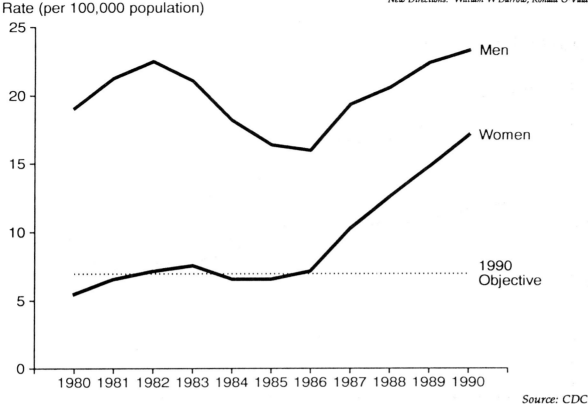

Source: CDC

Figure 5: Primary and secondary syphilis: rates by gender, United States, 1980-90, and 1990 objective.

Evaluation

We support efforts to evaluate the effectiveness and efficiency of planned interventions. However, we want to discourage evaluations that set out to determine if a single intervention delivered in one whopping dose results in permanent behaviour change, or if one intervention should completely replace another. Instead, we want to encourage evaluations in the 1990s that attempt to create programmes containing the most effective and efficient *combinations* of interventions. Some interventions should work better in some situations and with some populations than others, but most desirable are evaluations that determine how all available interventions combine to complement one another in maximising behaviour change and minimising the incidence of HIV and other STDs.

In the red-light district of Amsterdam, prostitutes who will only accept clients who agree to use condoms provide very effective information and education when they place a sticker saying "Ik doe het met" ("I do it with") in their windows. However, in Amsterdam and elsewhere, many prostitutes meet clients while walking the streets in certain parts of town. Counselling and voluntary testing for HIV antibodies and other STDs may be an effective way of making street prostitutes and their clients aware of their risks of HIV/STD infection and their HIV/STD infection status.

Several studies indicate that persons at risk for HIV/STD have difficulty talking with their sex partners about AIDS and other untoward consequences of unprotected sexual intercourse. Some people can tell their sex or needle-sharing partners that they have AIDS or are infected with HIV or other STDs. However, many do not want to know if they are infected or, if infected, they may want to conceal this fact. Post-test counselling and partner notification services are offered to those who are infected with HIV and other STDs to help them warn others about the dangers of unknowingly passing HIV and other agents to unprotected sex partners and their unborn children. Programmes must also arrange for infected persons to receive treatment and appropriate care, to be protected from stigmatisation and discrimination, and to be referred for other medical and social services. A major question facing us in the 1990s is, *"What is the optimal combination of activities and services we can provide to promote sexual health and prevent disease with the limited resources available to us?"*

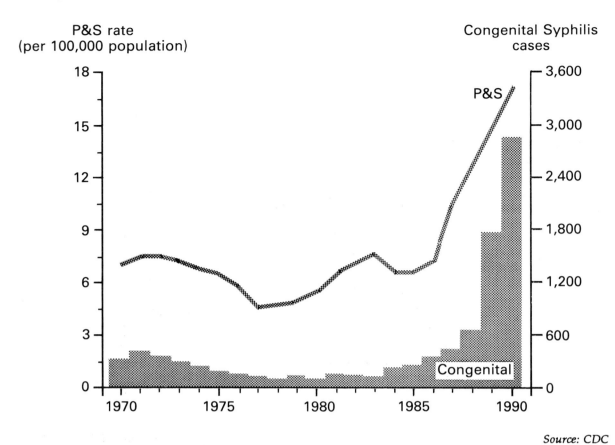

Source: CDC

Figure 6: Congenital syphilis: reported cases in infants <1 year of age and rates of primary and secondary syphilis in women: United States, 1970-90. (Note: case definition for congenital syphilis changed in 1989.)

Table 1: Proportion of never-married men aged 17-19 living in metropolitan areas of the USA who reported ever having had sexual intercourse

Year	White (%)	Black (%)	Total (%)
1979	64.5	71.1	65.7
1988	73.0	87.7	75.5

Source: Refs 11 and 12.

Table 2: Proportion of sexually active unmarried men aged 17-19 who reported using a condom at last sexual intercourse

Year	White and Hispanic (%)	Black (%)	Total (%)
1979	20.5	23.2	21.1
1988	56.5	62.0	57.5

Source: Refs 11 and 12.

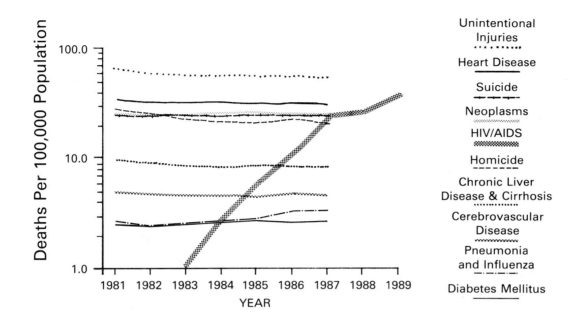

Data source: NCHS, CID.
Figure 7: Death rates for HIV/AIDS and other leading causes in men 25-44 years of age, United States, 1981-89.

Summary and Conclusions

To summarise, the five new directions for health promotion we have proposed for the 1990s are:

1. As an alternative to the "blunt instrument" of mass media information and education described by Jonathan Mann in London 1988, we recommend scalpel-sharp targetted messages, developed, implemented and reassessed by (or with) persons at greatest risk for HIV infection (or transmission) and with the realisation that health promotion is a multi-faceted, continuing process that should lead people through a series of steps towards permanent behavioural change.

2. As a remedy for disjointed efforts that are incapable of demonstrating impact or outcome, we recommend carefully designed programmes that implement interventions based on assessments of the problem and created to demonstrate incremental progress towards the goal of lowering the "reproductive rate" of HIV and other STDs.

3. As a cure for isolated efforts developed *de novo*, we recommend coordinated, comparative programmes that place interventions in context and test principles common to human beings interacting in social systems.

4. Because of limited resources, we cautiously recommend integration of activities and services to encourage efficiency of effort and to foster sound health decision-making in general.

5.   Finally, we recommend evaluation studies designed to determine the most effective and efficient blend of activities and services.

However, one obvious component missing in this logical model for health promotion in the 1990s is the human element of "affect" or emotion. As scientists, we are taught to react to data, but as human beings, we must not forget to react to our feelings. Thomas Parran made this point in his concluding chapter about the status of syphilis in Western societies in the 1930s[14]. He wrote:

> *"There are two great problems in public health: the first is the achievement of generalisation. Too frequently we judge the state of the nation by the single sector of it we see ourselves. In all public action, we cannot retain our sense of proportion unless we are supplied with facts enabling us to see things as a whole.*
>
> *"Public health workers have been so completely convinced of the necessity of generalisation, have so scorned the sentimental approach, that sometimes the need to be met seemed a problem in abstract statistics rather than one of flesh and blood. For this reason a second, and perhaps greatest need in the public health movement is the achievement of personalisation. We must be able to visualise the ascending death rate in terms of a man, a woman, a family. We must translate prevalence statistics into the terminology of pain."*

By 1989, AIDS was the second leading cause of death in men in the United States between the ages of 25 and 44 years (figure 7). This death rate has meaning to many of us because of our personal experiences with men we met and knew who were diagnosed with AIDS in the early 1980s. Other cases have come to our attention more recently through Mary Jane Edwards and an organisation she started called "Mothers of AIDS Patients". Mary Jane's son, Greg, was born in McAllen, Texas, in 1949; he was voted "most handsome" at Meadowbrook High School in Fort Worth, where he also excelled in swimming and diving, and won a scholarship to study the arts in New York City. While there, he became infected with HIV before anyone knew enough about AIDS to convince him to practise safer sex.

When Greg became so ill he could no longer care for himself, he returned to California. His mother tried to make his last days as meaningful as she could, but neither she nor anyone else could nurse him back to health. In her letter to me of September 22 1987, she wrote, *"Thank you for having an interest in my son, he was a wonderful person, my only child, and the light of my life."*

Greg is one of the 104,874 men, women and children in the United States who have died from AIDS. His mother wants everyone to know how much she misses her son, and how much she wants sexually active people throughout the world to minimise their risks of acquiring the virus that causes AIDS. When Mary Jane Edwards and other mothers of people with AIDS speak about how AIDS has changed their lives, everyone listens.

References

1. Mann J. Global AIDS: epidemiology, impact, projections, global strategy. *In* AIDS prevention and control. Oxford: Pergamon, 1988, 3-13.

2. Dawson D A, Cynamon M. AIDS knowledge and attitudes — provisional data from the national health interview survey: United States, August 1987. Advance Data from Vital and Health Statistics 1988; **146**: 1-12. (DHHS No. (PHS)88-1250)

3. Hardy A M. AIDS knowledge and attitudes for October-December 1989: provisional data from the national health interview survey. Advance Data from Vital and Health Statistics; No 186. Hyattsville MD: National Center for Health Statistics, 1990.

4. Prochaska J O, DiClemente C C. Toward a comprehensive model of change. *In* Miller W, Heather N (eds). Treating addictive behaviours. New York: Plenum, 1986, 3-27.

5. Alexander P. Prostitutes prevent AIDS: a manual for health educators. San Francisco: California Prostitutes Education Project, 1989.

6. Anderson R M, May R M. Epidemiological parameters of HIV transmission. Nature 1988; **333**: 514-9.

7. Brandt A M. No magic bullet: a social history of venereal disease in the United States since 1880. New York: Oxford Press, 1985.

8. Brandt A M. AIDS in historical perspective: four lessons from the history of sexually transmitted diseases. Am J Public Health 1988; **78**: 367-71.

9. Brandt A M. The syphilis epidemic and its relation to AIDS. Science 1988; **239**: 375-80.

10. Thomas G, Morgan-Witts M. Anatomy of an epidemic. Garden City NY: Doubleday, 1982.

11. Zelnik M, Kantner J F. Sexual activity, contraceptive use and pregnancy among metropolitan area teenagers: 1971-1979. Fam Plann Perspect 1980; **12**: 230-37.

12. Sonenstein F L, Pleck J H, Ku L C. Sexual activity, condom use and AIDS awareness among adolescent males. Fam Plann Perspect 1989; **21**: 152-58.

13. Forrest J D, Singh S. The sexual and reproductive behavior of American women, 1982-1988. Fam Plann Perspectives 1990; **22**: 206-14.

14. Parran T. Shadow on the land: syphilis. New York: Reynal and Hitchcock, 1937, 309.

Bibliography

Allen J R. Heterosexual transmission of human immunodeficiency virus (HIV) in the United States. Bull NY Acad Med 1988; **64**: 464-79.

Anderson R M, Cox D R, Hillier H C. Epidemiological and statistical aspects of the AIDS epidemic: introduction. Phil Trans R Soc Lond B 1989; **325**: 39-44.

Anderson R M, Blythe S P, Gupta S, Konings E. The transmission dynamics of the human immunodeficiency virus type 1 in the male homosexual community in the United Kingdom: the influence of changes in sexual behaviour. Phil Trans R Soc Lond B 1989; **325**: 45-98.

Anonymous. AIDS advertising campaign: report on four surveys during the first year of advertising — 1986-87. London: British Market Research Bureau Ltd, 1987.

Aral S O, Holmes K K. Sexually transmitted diseases in the AIDS era. Scientific American 1991; **264**: 62-9.

Ball J C, Lange W R, Myers C P, Friedman S R. Reducing the risk of AIDS through methadone maintenance treatment. J Health Soc Behavior 1988; **29**: 214-60.

Bauman L J, Siegel K. Misperceptions among gay men of the risk for AIDS associated with their sexual behavior. J Applied Social Psychol 1987; **17**: 329-50.

Baumgartner L, Curtis A C, Gray A L, Kuechle B E, Richman T L. The eradication of syphilis: a task report to the surgeon general public health service on syphilis control in the United States. Washington DC: US Government Printing Office, 1962. (Public Health Service Publication No. 918).

Bayer R. Private acts, social consequences: AIDS and the politics of public health. New York: Free Press, 1989.

Becker M H, Joseph J G. AIDS and behavioral change to reduce risk: a review. Am J Public Health 1988; **78**: 394-410.

Berk R A. Anticipating the social consequences of AIDS: a position paper. American Sociologist 1987; **18**: 211-41.

Burton S W, Burn S B, Harvey D, Mason M, McKerrow G. AIDS information. Lancet 1986; **2**: 1040-1.

Bye L. Designing an effective AIDS prevention campaign strategy for San Francisco: results from the first probability sample of an urban gay male community. San Francisco: Research and Decisions Corporation, 1984.

Campbell M J, Waters W E. Public knowledge about AIDS increasing. Br Med J 1987; **295**: 892-3.

Carne C A, Weller I V D, Johnson A M, et al. Prevalence of antibodies to human immunodeficiency virus, gonorrhoea rates and changed sexual behaviour in homosexual men in London. Lancet 1987; **1**: 656-8.

Cates W. Acquired immunodeficiency syndrome, sexually transmitted diseases, and epidemiology: past lessons, present knowledge, and future opportunities. Am J Epidemiol 1990; **131**: 749-58.

Cates W, Handsfield H H. HIV counseling and testing: does it work? Am J Public Health 1988; **78**: 1533-4.

Centers for Disease Control. Prevention of acquired immunodeficiency syndrome (AIDS): report of inter-agency recommendations. MMWR 1983; **32**: 101-4.

Centers for Disease Control. Declining rates of rectal and pharyngeal gonorrhea among males — New York City. MMWR 1984; **33**: 295-7.

Centers for Disease Control. Self-reported behavior change among gay and bisexual men — San Francisco. MMWR 1985; **34**: 613-5.

Centers for Disease Control. Additional recommendations to reduce sexual and drug abuse-related transmission of human T-lymphotropic virus type III/lymphadenopathy-associated virus. MMWR 1986; **35**: 152-5.

Centers for Disease Control. Self-reported changes in sexual behaviors among homosexual and bisexual men from the San Francisco city clinic cohort. MMWR 1987; **36**: 1987-9.

Centers for Disease Control. Guidelines for effective school health education to prevent the spread of AIDS. MMWR 1988; **37**, **S-2**: 1-14.

Centers for Disease Control. Condoms for prevention of sexually transmitted diseases. MMWR 1988; **37**: 133-7.

Centers for Disease Control. Understanding AIDS: an information brochure being mailed to all US households. MMWR 1988; **37**: 261-9.

Centers for Disease Control. Partner notification for preventing human immunodeficiency virus (HIV) infection — Colorado, Idaho, South Carolina, Virginia. MMWR 1988; **37**: 393-402.

Centers for Disease Control. Number of sex partners and potential risk of sexual exposure to human immunodeficiency virus. MMWR 1988; **37**: 565-8.

Centers for Disease Control. HIV infection reporting — United States. MMWR 1989; **38**: 496-9.

Centers for Disease Control. CDC plan for preventing human immunodeficiency virus (HIV) infection: a blueprint for the 1990s. Atlanta, GA: Centers for Disease Control, 1990. (HIV/ODD/1-90/001)

Chase A. Magic shots: a human and scientific account of the long and continuing struggle to eradicate infectious diseases by vaccination. New York: Morrow, 1982.

Check W A. Beyond the political model of reporting: nonspecific symptoms in media communications about AIDS. Rev Infect Dis 1987; **9**: 987-1000.

City and County of San Francisco, Department of Public Health. Rectal gonorrhea in San Francisco, October 1984-September 1986. San Francisco Epidemiologic Bulletin 1986; **2**: 1-3.

Colgate S A, Stanley E A, Hyman J M, Qualls C R, Layne S P. AIDS and a risk-based model. Los Alamos Science 1989; **18**: 2-39.

Communication Technologies. Designing an effective AIDS prevention campaign strategy for San Francisco: results from the fourth probability sample of an urban gay male community. San Francisco: Communication Technologies, 1987.

Coyle S L, Boruch R F, Turner C F, eds. Evaluating AIDS prevention programs: expanded edition. Washington DC: National Academy Press, 1991.

Darrow W W. Social and behavioral aspects of sexually transmitted diseases. *In*: Gordon S, Libby R W, eds. Sexuality today and tomorrow. North Scituate MA: Duxbury, 1976: 134-54.

Darrow W W. Approaches to the problem of venereal disease prevention. Prev Medicine 1976; **5**: 165-75.

Darrow W W. Social and psychological aspects of the sexually transmitted disease: a different view. Cutis 1981; **27**: 307-16.

Darrow W W. Sexual behavior in America: implications for the control of sexually transmitted diseases. *In*: Felman Y M, ed. Sexually transmitted diseases. New York: Churchill Livingstone, 1986: 261-80.

Darrow W W. A framework for preventing AIDS. Am J Public Health 1987; **77**: 778-9.

Darrow W W. Behavioral research and AIDS prevention. Science 1988; **239**: 1477.

DeGruttola V, Mayer K, Bennett W. AIDS: has the problem been adequately assessed? Rev Infect Dis 1986; **8**: 295-305.

Doll L S, Bye L L. AIDS: where reason prevails .... World Health Forum 1987; **8**: 484-8.

Dubois-Arber F, Lehmann P, Hausser D, Gutzwiller F, Zimmermann. Evaluation of the Swiss preventive campaigns against AIDS: second assessment report. Lausanne: Institut universitaire de medicine social et preventive, 1989. (Cah rech doc IUMSP No. 39b)

Fineberg H V. Education to prevent AIDS: prospects and obstacles. Science 1988; **239**: 592-6.

Foster S J, Furley K E. Public awareness survey on AIDS and condoms in Uganda. AIDS 1989; **3**: 147-54.

Francis D P, Chin J. The prevention of acquired immunodeficiency syndrome in the United States: an objective strategy for medicine, public health, business and the community. JAMA 1987; **257**: 1357-66.

Francis D P, Anderson R E, Gorman M E, et al. Targetting AIDS prevention and treatment toward HIV-1 infected persons: the concept of early intervention. JAMA 1989; **262**: 2572-6.

Freudenberg N. Preventing AIDS: a guide to effective education for the prevention of HIV infection. Washington DC: American Public Health Association, 1989.

Gamson J. Silence, death, and the invisible enemy: AIDS activism and social movement "newness". Social Problems 1989; **36**: 351.

Goedert J J. What is safe sex? N Eng J Med 1987; **316**: 1339-42.

Gordon R. A critical review of the physics and statistics of condoms and their role in the individual versus societal survival of the AIDS epidemic. J Sex Marital Therapy 1989; **15**: 5-30.

Gostin L O. Public health strategies for confronting AIDS: legislative and regulatory policy in the United States. JAMA 1989; **261**: 1621-30.

Green L W, Lewis F M. Measurement and evaluation in health education and health promotion. Palo Alto CA: Mayfield, 1986.

Hastings G B, Leather D S, Scott A C. AIDS publicity: some experiences from Scotland. Br Med J 1987; **294**: 48-9.

Hausser D, Lehmann P, Dubois-Arber F, Gutzwiller F. Evaluation des campagnes de prevention contr le SIDA en Suisse. Lausanne: Institut universitaire de medicine sociale et preventive, 1987. (Cah rech doc IUMSP No 23)

Hearst N, Hulley S B. Preventing the heterosexual spread of AIDS: are we giving our patients the best advice? JAMA 1988; **259**: 2426-32.

Institute of Medicine, National Academy of Sciences. Mobilizing against AIDS: the unfinished story of a virus. Cambridge MA: Harvard University Press, 1986.

Job R F S. Effective and ineffective use of fear in health promotion campaigns. Am J Public Health 1988; **78**: 163-7.

Johnson A M. Social and behavioural aspects of the HIV epidemic: a review. J R Statist Soc A 1988; **151, part 1**: 99-114.

Johnson A M, Gill O N. Evidence of recent changes in sexual behaviour in homosexual men in England and Wales. Phil Trans R Soc Lond B 1989; **325**: 153-61.

Jones C C, Waskin H, Gerety B, et al. Persistence of high-risk sexual activity among homosexual men in an area of low incidence of the acquired immunodeficiency syndrome. Sex Transm Dis 1987; **14**: 17-20.

Joseph J G, Montgomery S B, Emmons C A, et al. Magnitude and determinants of behavioral risk reduction: longitudinal analysis of a cohort at risk for AIDS. Psychology and Health 1987; **1**: 73-96.

Kahn J R, Kalsbeek W D, Hofferth S L. National estimates of teenage sexual activity; evaluating the comparability of three national surveys. Demography 1988; **25**: 189-204.

Kaplan E H, Abramson P R. So what if the program ain't perfect: a mathematical model of AIDS education. Evaluation Review 1989; **13**: 107-22.

Kaplan H B, Johnson R J, Bailey C A, Simon W. The sociological study of AIDS; a critical review of the literature and suggested research agenda. J Health Soc Behavior 1987; **28**: 140-57.

Kaplan J E, Spira T, Fishbein D. Reasons for decrease in sexual activity in homosexual men with HIV infection. JAMA 1988; **260**: 2836-7.

Kelly J A, St Lawrence J S. The AIDS health crisis: psychological and social interventions. New York: Plenum, 1988.

Kelly J A, St Lawrence J S, Hood H V, Brasfield T L. Behavioral intervention to reduce AIDS risk activities. Jour Consult Clin Psychol 1989; **57**: 60-7.

Kelly J A, St Lawrence J S. Behavioral group intervention to teach AIDS risk reduction skills. Jackson MS: University of Mississippi Medical Center, 1990.

Kelly J A, St Lawrence J S, Brasfield T L, Stevenson L Y, Dias Y E, Hauth A C. AIDS risk behavior patterns among gay men in small Southern cities. Am J Public Health 1990; **80**: 416-18.

Kotarba J A. Ethnography and AIDS. J Contemp Ethnography 1990; **19**: 259-70.

Kuller L H, Kingsley L A. The epidemic of AIDS: the failure of public health policy. Millbank Quarterly 1986; **64, suppl. 1**: 56-78.

Lehmann P, Hausser D, Somaini B, Gutzwiller F. Campaign against AIDS in Switzerland: evaluation of a nationwide educational programme. Br Med J 1987; **295**: 1118-20.

Lisken L, Blackburn R, Maier J H. AIDS — a public health crisis. Population Reports 1986; **14**: L193-L228.

Mason J O. CDC and STD: evolving roles. Proceedings — 1988 STD national conference. Atlanta GA: Centers for Disease Control, 1988: 1-3.

Mason J O, Noble G R, Lindsey B K, et al. Current CDC efforts to prevent and control human immunodeficiency virus infection and AIDS in the United States. Public Health Rep 1988; **103**: 255-60.

Masters W J, Johnson V E, Kolodny R C. Crisis: heterosexual behavior in the age of AIDS. New York: Grove, 1988.

Matthews G W, Neslund V S. The initial impact of AIDS on public health law in the United States — 1986. JAMA 1987; **257**: 344-52.

Mays V M, Cochran S D. Issues in the perception of AIDS risk and risk reduction activities by black and hispanic/latina women. American Psychologist 1988; **43**: 949-57.

MsKusick L, Conant M, Coates T J. The AIDS epidemic: a model for developing intervention strategies for reducing high-risk behavior in gay men. Sex Transm Dis 1985; **12**: 229-34.

McKusick L, Wiley J A, Coates T J, et al. Reported changes in the sexual behavior of men at risk for AIDS, San Francisco, 1982-84 — the AIDS behavioral research project. Public Health Rep 1985; **100**: 622-9.

Miller H G, Turner C F, Moses L E, eds. AIDS: the second decade. Washington DC: National Academy Press, 1990.

Mills S, Campbell M J, Waters W E. Public knowledge of AIDS and the DHSS advertisement campaign. Br Med J 1986; **293**: 1089-90.

Nelkin D. AIDS and the social sciences: review of useful knowledge and research needs. Rev Infect Dis 1987; **9**: 980-6.

Ngugi E. Bringing the programme to the audience. AIDS Health Promotion Exchange 1988; **2**: 5.

Ngugi E N, Plummer F A, Simonsen J N, et al. Prevention of transmission of human immunodeficiency virus in Africa: effectiveness of condom promotion and health education among prostitutes. Lancet 1988; **2**: 887-90.

O'Reilly, K R, Higgins D L. The AIDS community demonstration projects: a multicenter community based research. Public Health Rep (in press).

Osborn J E. AIDS: politics and science. N Engl J Med 1988; **318**: 444-7.

Perlman J A, Kelaghan J, Wolf P H, Baldwin W, Coulson A, Novello A. HIV risk difference between condom users and nonusers among US heterosexual women. J Acquir Immune Deficiency Syndromes 1990; **3**: 155-65.

Reiss I L, Leik R K. Evaluating strategies to avoid AIDS: number of partners vs. use of condoms. J Sex Research 1989; **26**: 411-33.

Rugg D L, MacGowan R J, Stark K A, Swanson N M. An evaluation challenge: HIV counseling and testing. Public Health Rep (in press).

St Lawrence J S, Hood H V, Brasfield T, Kelly J A. Differences in gay men's AIDS risk knowledge and behavior patterns in high and low AIDS prevalence cities. Public Health Rep 1989; **104**: 391-5.

Searle E S. Knowledge, attitudes and behaviour of health professionals in relation to AIDS. Lancet 1987; **1**: 26-8.

Seltzer V L, Rabin J, Benjamin F. Teenagers' awareness of the acquired immunodeficiency syndrome and the impact on their sexual behavior. Obstet Gynecol 1989; **74**: 55-9.

Sherr L. Fear arousal and AIDS: do shock tactics work? AIDS 1990; **4**: 361-4.

Shikles J L. AIDS education: issues affecting counseling and testing programs. Washington DC: General Accounting Office, 1989.

Shilts R. And the band played on: politics, people and the AIDS epidemic. New York: St Martin's Press, 1987.

Siegel K, Grodsky P B, Herman A. AIDS risk-reducing guidelines: a review and analysis. J Community Health 1986; **11**: 233-43.

Siegel K, Baumann L J, Christ G H, Krown S. Patterns of change in sexual behavior among gay men in New York City. Arch Sex Behavior 1988; **17**: 481-97.

Siegel K, Glassman M. Individual and aggregate level change in sexual behavior among gay men at risk for AIDS. Arch Sex Behavior 1989; **18**: 335-48.

Siegel K, Levine M P, Brooks C, Kern R. The motives of gay men for taking or not taking the HIV antibody test. Social Problems 1989; **36**: 368-83.

Siegel K, Mesagno F P, Chen J Y, Grace C. Factors distinguishing homosexual males practicing risky and safer sex. Soc Sci Med 1989; **28**: 561-9.

Singer E, Rogers T F. Public opinion and AIDS. AIDS and Public Policy Journal 1986; **1**: 8-13.

Singer E, Rogers T F, Corcoran M. The polls — a report: AIDS. Pub Opinion Quarterly 1987; **51**: 80-95.

Sisk J E, Hewitt M, Metcalf K L. The effectiveness of AIDS education. Health Affairs 1988; **7**: 37-51.

Skidmore C A, Robertson J R, Robertson A A, Elton R A. After the epidemic: follow up study of HIV seroprevalence and changing patterns of drug use. Br Med J 1990; **300**: 219-23.

Smith T W. Adult sexual behavior in 1989: number of partners, frequency of intercourse and risk of AIDS. Fam Plann Perspect 1991; **23(3)**: 102-7.

Staub R. The Swiss hot rubber campaign. AIDS Health Promotion Exchange 1988; **2**: 6-7.

Turner C F, Miller H G, Moses L E, eds. AIDS, sexual behavior, and intravenous drug use. Washington DC: National Academy Press, 1989.

Udry J R, Clark L T, Chase C L, Levy M. Can mass media advertising increase contraceptive use? Fam Plann Perspectives 1972; **4**: 37-44.

US Congress, Office of Technology Assessment. How effective is AIDS education? Washington DC: US Government Printing Office, 1988.

US Dept of Health and Human Services, Public Health Service. Coolfont report: a PHS plan for prevention and control of AIDS and the AIDS virus. Public Health Rep 1986; **101**: 341-8.

US General Accounting Office. AIDS education: reaching populations at higher risk. Gaithersburg MD: US Government Printing Office, 1988. (Document No GAO/PEMD-88-35)

Valdiserri R O. Preventing AIDS: the design of effective programs. New Brunswick NJ: Rutgers, 1989.

Watkins J D, Conway-Welch C, Creedon J J, et al. Interim report of the presidential commission on the human immunodeficiency virus epidemic: chairman's recommendations — part 1. J Acquir Immune Deficiency Syndromes 1988; **1**: 69-103.

Wellings K, Field J, Wadsworth J, Johnson A M, Anderson R M, Bradshaw S A. Sexual lifestyles under scrutiny. Nature 1990; **348**: 276-8.

The Economics of Promoting Sexual Health

Christine Godfrey, Keith Tolley and Michael Drummond
Centre for Health Economics,
University of York

(Oral presentation by Mrs Godfrey)

Abstract

Economists have taken a lead in estimating the potential costs of the spread of HIV infection. These estimates of the resource implications have stimulated the policy debate about the need for preventive policies. While the resources devoted to prevention may seem small compared to the potential costs of AIDS and other sexually transmitted diseases, it is still important to ensure that all resources are used cost effectively. The main purpose of this paper is to outline the economist's perspective and its applicability to the choice of strategies for promoting sexual health.

Economic evaluation techniques involve measuring both the costs and benefits of health programmes, which can be assessed from different viewpoints. Evaluating health promotion activities in general, and those promoting sexual health in particular, poses a number of challenges. For example, it is unclear to what extent health promotion has been responsible for changes in behaviour in some homosexual communities. Furthermore, while some information is available about the rates of new AIDS cases, a lack of accurate data makes it impossible to determine the true rate of new cases of HIV infection. The lack of specific evidence has limited the use of formal economic evaluation. It is, however, possible to examine the range of alternative strategies for promoting sexual health and the features of the policy alternatives which may affect the balance between costs and benefits. In this way the advantages of an economic perspective can be explored and priorities for co-ordinating and structuring research using a number of different perspective outlined.

Introduction

Economists have taken a lead in estimating the potential costs of the spread of HIV infection[1,2,3]. These estimates of the resource implications have stimulated the policy debate about the need for preventive policies. Many countries have funded a wide range of different initiatives for the primary and secondary prevention of HIV infection and other sexually transmitted diseases. While the resources devoted to prevention may seem small compared to the potential costs of the disease, it is still important to ensure that all resources are used cost effectively. Therefore, economists are beginning to address the questions of evaluating alternative prevention strategies[4].

The main purpose of this paper is to outline the economist's perspective and its applicability to the choice of strategies for promoting sexual health. In the first section of the paper some key economic concepts are discussed. The use of these concepts to consider the balance of costs and benefits attached to both primary and secondary prevention of sexually transmitted diseases is explored in the second section of the paper. Finally some conclusions are drawn on how the economist's perspective can be developed to aid the difficult choices facing authorities dealing with the consequences of HIV/AIDS and other sexually transmitted diseases.

Key Economic Concepts

Opportunity cost

One of the most important economic concepts is that of *opportunity cost*. Economics starts from the premise that resources are scarce and the opportunity cost of using a given resource is the benefits that could be obtained from using it in its best alternative use. This concept is particularly important when discussing emotive issues such as the spread of HIV/AIDS since there may be a tendency to argue that resources should be made freely available to combat the epidemic. However, all resources have an opportunity cost and when more resources are devoted to HIV/AIDS something else is being given up, either within other fields of health care or in the economy more generally. Moreover, this concept carries the implication that using resources inefficiently is unethical since benefits elsewhere are unnecessarily forgone[5].

Types of costs and benefits

Economic evaluations identify, measure and value the costs and benefits attached to a number of alternative policies. The comparison of these costs and benefits is used to identify those policies that yield the highest net benefits, based upon the opportunity cost principle. The alternatives considered can include "doing nothing" and for sexually transmitted diseases this alternative is not costless. The relevance of an economic evaluation to inform policy choices will partially depend on which policies are considered. Some of the different questions that could be addressed in this field include: are resources being devoted to HIV/AIDS or other STDs giving value for money compared to other health and social care; is the balance of funds between prevention, treatment and research correct; what should be the priorities within the prevention budget? Answering these questions can involve the use of different types of economic evaluation. *Cost-benefit analysis* involves the identification and valuation of all the relevant costs and benefits of alternative prevention programmes. In contrast, *cost-effectiveness analysis* uses a single uniform measure of benefit to compare alternative programmes. The alternative uses of different forms of economic evaluations for AIDS/HIV are explored in more detail in Godfrey and Tolley[6].

Costs and benefits can be divided into three main categories: direct; indirect; and intangible. Direct costs of prevention programmes should be the easiest items to identify but, surprisingly very few estimates are given in the literature. Direct health benefits arising from prevention activities are the avoided mortality, morbidity and health service use from changes in the rates of sexually transmitted diseases. Campaigns which stress positive aspects of safer sexual practices may have additional benefits in improving quality of life as well as preventing ill-health.

Most prevention activities have a number of broader effects. For example, those attending special clinics or or screening tests may have travelling expenses and the time attending a clinic or undertaking a health education activity has some "cost" in lost working or leisure time. While the benefits of health promotion and prevention activities have been mainly considered in terms of gains in health status, there may be other, non-health, benefits. For example, some argue that information gained from health promotion activities has a value whether behaviour is changed or not[7].

Hence, with the provision of better information on risks, individuals can make more informed choices about their sexual behaviour and therefore a component of the economic benefit is the value individuals place on this additional information. It is likely that this value will vary between groups and across cultures.

Most of the existing economic studies of HIV/AIDS concentrate on the direct health care costs and the consequences in terms of productivity losses[2]. Since AIDS affects people at a relatively young age the losses in production can be as much as five times the size of direct heath care costs. Whilst this approach gives high estimates of the economic costs of AIDS/HIV, some economists have concerns about its validity[1]. An alternative approach would be to assess the consequences of disease in terms of its impact on length and quality of life. Not all sexually transmitted diseases are life-threatening and impacts on quality of life are therefore important.

In most health care evaluations no attempt is made to value the intangible costs and benefits, although they may be identified. Pain and anxiety are associated with a number of different prevention activities relating to sexual behaviour and it may therefore be important to attempt to evaluate the level of these intangible items between programmes. For example, some programmes may reduce anxiety for some, but if poorly targeted increase anxiety and create "worried well".

Differing viewpoints

The economic costs and benefits of prevention programmes can be assessed from different viewpoints. A particular course of action may be judged as cost-effective from the viewpoint on one group, say the health authority or agency providing the programme, but not be cost-effective for society as a whole. In general economists advocate that evaluations should be considered from a societal viewpoint and for HIV/AIDS this is particularly important as many costs and benefits are incurred by individuals and agencies such as voluntary bodies outside the health care sector. In addition, changing the risky behaviour of one individual has benefits to third parties by limiting the spread of disease. (These are known, in economic terms, as *external benefits* or *externalities*.) The benefits of encouraging those with the virus to modify sexual behaviour will accrue mainly to those individuals' potential sexual partners and to society as a whole if the spread of the virus is contained. The infected individual may gain very little.

The presence of external benefits is in contrast to other campaigns to change behaviour, such as dietary change, where the main health benefits are individually based. This has implications for the choice of outcomes measures to compare alternative prevention programmes. Measures such as "informed person" or "needles exchanged" may be inadequate if external benefits not included in these measures are likely to vary between programmes.

Although economists would advocate a broad social viewpoint when considering the overall cost-effectiveness of different programmes, additional insights can be gained from considering costs and benefits from different viewpoints within the evaluation process. In particular, there is a need to consider the complex array of incentives and disincentives encountered by individuals engaging in sexual relationships. Birch and Stoddart[8] outline an economic model of individual choices of sexual behaviour. The main prediction of this model is that some individuals, in identifying, measuring, valuing and comparing the perceived costs and benefits of different behaviour, may decide that continuing risky behaviour is in their own best interest. However, the authors suggest that these individual decisions are strongly influenced by a number of societal and environmental factors. For example, education and experience will determine the individual perceptions of the nature and size of benefits and costs of different patterns of sexual behaviour. Also expectations of future income and social support will influence the values put on perceived costs and benefits. The emerging links between poverty and HIV/AIDS have already been noted as a cause for concern.

Another factor influencing the values put on different costs and benefits is variations in attitudes towards risk. O'Brien[9] discusses the relevance of studying risk assessment in relation to HIV/AIDS. A distinction is often made in the literature between objective and subjective risks. Behaviour may be modified because perceived risks are higher than actual risks. In the case of HIV/AIDS this may be seen as desirable if the transmission of the virus is reduced. However, extreme precautionary behaviour may not be without its own costs or disbenefits and may be linked to stigma of those with the virus. Also, to be effective, behaviour change will need to be permanent. There is danger that, in reaction to the slow down in new AIDS cases, behavioural change may be reversed. Such shifts in behaviour in reaction to changing perceived risks are not unknown in other areas. For example, the introduction of roadside breath tests in the UK was initially very successful in reducing the numbers of drinking drivers. However, when it was realised that the probability of being breathalysed was low, drivers reverted to old patterns of drinking and driving[10]. A major implication of economic models is that attention needs to be placed on the costs and benefits facing key actors and the incentives that might need to be put in place to change their behaviour.

Uncertainty in costs and benefits

There is considerable uncertainty about current numbers of people who are HIV positive and the forecasts of both the future incidence and costs associated with the problem. The lack of basic epidemiological data has been blamed for the wide range of predictions and there have been political problems in both the UK and US in funding general surveys of sexual behaviour[11,12]. Wide ranges of treatment costs have also been presented in the literature. Scitovsky[13] cites a number of factors affecting the estimates of treatment costs. The estimates of cost per treated person have fallen considerably over time but changes in available treatments may lead to an increase in the proportion of those HIV+ receiving treatment. Treatment costs have fallen partly though less aggressive management and lower doses of some drugs. Changes in the composition of the population with the disease and the diffusion of the epidemic from main population centres are given by Scitovsky as possible causes of increasing treatment costs per person in the future. Another factor influencing treatment costs is the price of drugs. However, if some drugs are more widely adopted for use in delaying the onset of AIDS, drug companies may be persuaded to lower prices further and better management may lower drug dosage[14].

Health care treatment costs are only one component of the total costs of AIDS/HIV. Tolley *et al*[15] give a range of figures for the costs of social care in the UK. In 1989 these costs were estimated to range from £17 per week as a low cost estimate of the social care for those HIV+ to £106 per week as a high estimate for those with AIDS. This includes the costs of informal care which on average was valued at £19 a week. There are uncertainties, however, about the services which will be provided and the total uptake and mix of social and health care services will vary from country to country, depending in part on how services are funded[14].

Given the large number of uncertainties in estimating costs and benefits associated with HIV/AIDS, the usual approach, known as sensitivity analysis, may be inadequate. One development is the use of scenario analysis which has been advocated for the study of AIDS by Jager et al.[16] Scenario analysis requires modelling of all interactions between key variables. For AIDS this implies linking modelling of the probability of infection with the socio-cultural and economic impact of HIV/AIDS on society. The data requirements of building such models are considerable but, if successful, these studies could provide a useful tool in stimulating the effects of various prevention strategies.

Marginal analysis

Although some policy decisions relate to a simple choice between two or more alternatives, usually information is required on *how much* of a policy should be applied. For example, to answer questions on the extent of coverage of a prevention programme, or how many or how often screening tests should be given, requires the consideration of marginal costs and benefits; that is, exploration of the variation of costs and benefits with the size of the programme. Mulley *et al*[17], in a study of the use of the vaccine for Hepatitis B, investigated variations in cost-effectiveness of combinations of screening and vaccination for the whole population, compared with two groups who were identified as being at high risk from contracting the virus (homosexual men and surgical residents). Marginal costs and benefits did vary between the groups and the results suggested that screening followed by vaccination of homosexual men, and vaccination without prior screening of surgical residents, would result in savings of medical costs, but that neither screening nor vaccination would be the lowest cost strategy for the population as a whole.

Applications of Economic Concepts to Strategies for Promoting Sexual Health

Economic evaluations, if carried out with care, can provide useful guidance for policy makers. One approach would be to consider primary promotion and secondary prevention as alternative strategies that could be chosen for promoting sexual health. An overall objective for primary promotion may be to change individuals' behaviour to undertake safer sexual practices in order to reduce their risk of being infected with HIV or any other STD. In contrast, a package of secondary prevention measures would be likely to focus on those who have the HIV virus in an attempt to minimise the risk of their spreading the infection to others. The costs and benefits involved in different potential components of a primary or a secondary prevention programme are considered separately below. In practice, alternative strategies are likely to involve a combination of primary and secondary measures, which makes the separation of the costs and benefits associated with each component more difficult. Some aspects of the choice of strategy in practice are considered in a third sub-section below.

Primary promotion

Most commentators[18,19,20] have expressed the view that changing behaviour through primary health promotion initiatives is the only means available to stop the spread of HIV/AIDS. Estimates of the cost of treatment are seen as one indicator of the potential benefits of prevention but there is little information on the other costs and benefits of prevention programmes. There is evidence that behaviour among some communities has been modified[21] but considerable difficulties have been encountered in linking these changes in behaviour to any specific interventions. Despite the recognition of the importance of prevention, and the initial funding of mass media campaigns in many countries, there is little evidence that funds for primary prevention are given priority when budgets are limited. (See, for example, Tolley and Maynard[22] for the position in the UK.)

In primary promotion it is particularly important to demonstrate that behavioural change will take place. For most STDs, including HIV, the changes in behaviour being sought are similar, but, as discussed above, they are likely to involve costs to the individual. Hence some prevention initiatives may be specifically targetted at reducing these costs by, for example, increasing the availability and acceptability of condoms, or developing skills to reduce the anxiety and embarrassment of initiating safer sex practices. The choice of the "message" or content of a campaign is one component of a prevention strategy needing evaluation. The economic approach, along with other models, would suggest that information about the risks of disease is only one option. Alternative approaches include messages which stress the positive aspects of safe sex or minimise the perceived costs of behavioural change. Campaigns based on creating "fear", or emphasising the perceived costs if infected, may not be the most effective approaches and can carry costs to those not at risk from infection.

Criticisms of messages in campaigns have mainly been directed at mass media campaigns where it can be difficult to be informative. Hence with such campaigns there is a risk of increasing anxiety of those at risk, and those with little risk, without providing the means of reassurance. The initial UK mass advertisement campaign was criticised[23] but later campaigns included a helpline number which was extensively used[24]. Generally evaluations of the UK and other mass publicity schemes have suggested that these have increased in knowledge but have been of limited use in changing behaviour[20]. Mass media and nationally based publicity campaigns are an expensive part of any preventive strategy. For example, the campaign to distribute a leaflet in every household in the UK was estimated to cost £20m[25]. In other fields of health education it has been argued that mass media campaigns should be seen to have the function of "agenda setting", supplying motivation or awareness of a health problem, rather than directly altering individual behaviour. However, Redman *et al*[26], in an extensive general review on the effectiveness of mass media campaigns, concluded ".. there is currently no evidence that the media component makes a major contribution to the effectiveness of such combined programmes. It may be that the community component presented alone or in combination with a cheaper method of agenda-setting can provide similar magnitude behaviour changes."

Community based programmes can also take many forms and one of the problems facing economic and other evaluations is separating out and comparing the cost-effectiveness of various components of programmes[27]. As in mass media campaigns there are alternative types of message which can be delivered. The information content and targetting of messages may be easier to achieve within a community based programme and may help to minimise costs and maximise benefits to individuals of changing behaviour. Examples of the different elements of such campaigns are given in Coates[21]. From an economic perspective there is a potential for inappropriate use of resources if there is duplication in the design of projects and the development of campaign material across communities. Therefore, exchange of information on the design and evaluation of materials is important. Similarly, there may be a cost saving potential in combining some HIV and STD programmes.

Within programmes there is also the choice of agency to deliver the health promotion message. Particular problems have been encountered in the field of promoting sexual health, as statutory bodies often have restrictions on the level of explicitness of their material, compared with that of voluntary agencies[21]. These problems suggest some trade-off between social morals and health for different groups in society. Economic evaluations do not provide a means of reconciling such trade-offs but are a means of making them explicit. Comprehensive community based programmes may include a number of agencies and sites including schools, workplaces, STD and family planning clinics and health care professionals. A large part of prevention expenditure on HIV/AIDS in the UK has been directed at educating professional groups, especially those within the health care system, who may in turn play a part in the health promotion process[20,28]. The effectiveness of this approach has not, however, been evaluated. Health Authorities in the UK have now been directed to spend at least £1.4m. of additional funds allocated in 1989/90 on "community based initiatives aimed at helping individuals change behaviour which puts them at risk of HIV infection"[29].

General Practitioners in the UK have not traditionally played a prominent role in the prevention of STDs. Rather, activity has been centred on specialised clinics. It might be argued that the economic advantage of using primary care physicians relates both to cost and compliance. Opportunistic screening and counselling involves fewer resources than specialised clinics. With patients already *in situ* and primary care physicians routinely seeing people who may not come forward to specific invitations, health promotion may be well targetted to those with risky behaviour. The choice between general and specialised settings is, however, far from resolved and available evidence suggests that people with HIV infection or AIDS prefer to receive support from specialised HIV workers[15].

A wide range of means of communication have been used in HIV/AIDS campaigns including telephone and postal campaigns[30]. Some advocate the advantages of personal contact to promote behavioural change[31]. A major factor affecting the cost of a campaign is the use of labour. However, whether the costs of specialised counselling is justified can only be assessed by comparing its effectiveness with other approaches. Intensive campaigns targetted at high risk groups, such as some outreach campaigns for prostitutes, have large potential benefits if behaviour is changed. The evidence for making choices between *diffuse* (but lower cost) campaigns, versus *targetted* (but resource intensive) programmes is not yet available.

Secondary prevention

While few economic evaluations have been undertaken for primary promotion activities there is a far larger general literature on the economics of secondary prevention[32]. One of the major distinctions between HIV/AIDS and other sexually transmitted diseases is the availability of effective therapies. The major impact of the success of different therapies will be on the benefits to individuals of undertaking a screening test. For some diseases earlier identification through screening will bring benefits in terms of improved prognosis, less radical treatment and avoided morbidity and mortality. In addition, whether treatment is effective or not, those individuals having true negative test results will benefit from reassurance. Other than such reassurance for some, at present the balance of costs and benefits for individuals to undertake an antibody test for HIV is still unclear. On the one hand identification will allow individuals to undergo therapy that may delay the onset of AIDS. On the other hand a responsible individual would have to change his or her lifestyle considerably after being identified as being HIV positive and carry the burden for longer.

For all sexually transmitted diseases there are *external* benefits from screening. Where therapies are available to cure the disease the screening process has the potential to affect directly the pool of disease and hence the risks to third parties. In some cases (such as syphilis or gonorrhoea) this has led to medical recommendations of epidemiological treatment, that is treatment at the presenting visit whether symptoms are present or not for "at risk" groups[33]. In this case the external benefits, in terms of disease prevention, are deemed (by the clinician) to outweigh the possible individual costs of toxic reaction to unneeded therapy. For other diseases where therapies do not cure the infection in the individual, external benefits will only be achieved if the individual changes behaviour. Screening programmes provide the opportunity to educate on safer behaviour irrespective of the test result. Some evidence does suggest that those diagnosed HIV+ adopt safer sexual practices[34]. In a study of 181 people in the UK with HIV/AIDS approximately 90 per cent of the respondents said they had made changes in their sexual lives since diagnosis[15]. However, it can not be expected that all identified HIV+ will change behaviour or that changes in behaviour will be the same across all groups.

Considerable attention has been given to the screening of women of child-bearing age for sexually transmitted diseases, because of the risk of transmission of disease in pregnancy. The benefits in this case are the avoided mortality and morbidity of the infants. In the UK there had been routine antenatal screening for syphilis. Williams[35] investigated the cost-effectiveness of this procedure. The benefits of the screening programme were measured in terms of the avoided resource costs of the health and educational needs of affected infants and the "pain and suffering" for the parents associated with excess stillbirths, neonatal deaths and the birth of a disabled child. Despite the low prevalence of syphilis this screening programme was judged to be cost-effective. There are a number of problems in evaluating antenatal screening because most benefits would only be achieved through abortion and such moral issues may be thought to be outside the economist's perspective[36]. Controversy surrounding the availability of abortions has limited the advice given in the US and other countries about routine screening for HIV in pregnant women. Recommendations have generally been limited to prenatal testing but that is only relevant for planned pregnancies. The costs and benefits to women in terms of reproductive rights are clearly complex[37].

The costs of screening can fall on the individual or society more generally. The distribution of costs depends on whether individuals are charged for screening, or whether the costs are covered by insurance or financed from state finances. Individuals, however, may bear additional costs. As well as the out-of-pocket expenses and loss of time incurred undertaking a screening test (and counselling) there are a number of intangible costs. These include embarrassment and anxiety. In the UK, because of life insurance rules there are a number of other costs associated with undertaking an HIV test. The Department of Health has sought changes to these rules in an attempt to lower these costs and to extend the take-up of voluntary testing, but with no apparent success[38].

Other costs to individuals will depend on the outcome of the screening test and the disease. Where individuals undertake treatment, as a result of the test, more cost will be imposed on the individual, although generally there will also be benefits. Individuals may not appreciate the benefits of treatment if their disease is asymptomatic. Where therapies are available the overall cost-effectiveness will depend on the compliance with treatment. For diseases with no current effective therapy a positive result can bring both considerable intangible costs and in some cases additional morbidity[34].

Different costs are borne by those with a false positive or false negative results. As well as genuine false negative results there is some concern that those with true negative results may react by continuing risky behaviour. False positive results may, however, be felt to impose the higher individual costs and this has led to recommendations against the widespread testing for HIV. The US Preventive Task Force quote figures that a screening test with high sensitivity and specificity of 99% will generate 10 false positives for every on case detected in a population with a prevalence of 0.1 per cent. Mandatory testing of individuals in low risk populations has proved ineffective in identifying those with the disease. No formal cost-benefit analysis has been carried out on general populations for HIV, but available evidence does tend to support the Task Force's recommendations.

More generally the direct costs of screening programmes will depend on the cost of the test, the numbers tested and for some diseases the increase in treatment costs that may result because of the screening programme. Another factor which may reduce indirect and intangible costs but increase direct costs is pre- and post-test counselling. While this has been recommended for HIV tests it is not always available. For example, in a survey of those HIV+ in the UK between 1983 and 1990, 61% received no pre-test counselling and 38% no post-test counselling, although rates of counselling increased the later the test had occurred[15].

For the economic evaluations of other screening programmes one factor influencing overall cost-effectiveness is the ability to target programmes at those most likely to benefit. For sexually transmitted diseases this has been attempted by carrying out tests at specialised clinics with some outreach programmes for those with risky behaviours. Outreach programmes can be expensive, especially on a per capita basis, and there is no clear evidence that even if those most at risk are targetted, that compliance with the aims of the screening programme, whether behaviour change or treatment, will be high enough to justify the additional funds.

Another factor influencing cost-effectiveness is the optimum timing of repeated screening. The need to repeat screening and other problems suggest that schemes to isolate those who are HIV+ would not be effective. In addition, they would impose very high costs on some individuals. At present in the UK testing is being undertaken on a voluntary basis although some groups with risk behaviour, for example drug users, have been targetted in publicity to volunteer for testing. It is not clear that the voluntary approach is the best use of resources as it may encourage some at low risk to be "over tested" while others at "high risk" may not come forward without more substantial campaigns.

Another secondary prevention activity is contact tracing and partner notification. These programmes have been thought to be successful for some sexually transmitted diseases[33] although information is not available to estimate the cost-effectiveness of this approach for HIV/AIDS.

Choice of Strategy

A key part of the economic evaluation of the promotion of healthy sexual behaviour involves the clarification of the main objectives of any policy, and the alternative strategies that could be used for achieving these objectives. The previous discussion has considered separately primary health promotion and secondary prevention. This distinction is useful as an illustration of the important issues facing the analyst in determining the potential costs and benefits of either approach considered in isolation. For sexually transmitted diseases other than HIV infection, alternative packages may exist based on either primary promotion, secondary prevention or no prevention. This is because effective treatments are available and so the potential costs of an absence of prevention are less severe but still sizeable for some diseases[34]. The evidence from economic evaluations of prevention programmes suggests that even where effective therapies exist, prevention is not always better than cure[39]. Ineffective or unproven prevention programmes are almost certainly a waste of scarce resources.

There are a number of factors that make the identification of clear cut alternative packages of primary promotion and secondary prevention difficult, especially for HIV infection. For example, HIV screening and testing (part of secondary prevention) may target all "at risk" individuals. Hence all those individuals who are tested as HIV negative may still receive "safer sex" health education (primary promotion) because of their "at risk" status. In practice, promoting sexual health will involve a variety of measures and the policy choice involves the mix of programme components. An important use for an economic evaluation is to examine the impact on costs and benefits of a change in the balance of the primary and secondary components of sexual health promotion packages.

The economist's perspective is also useful for evaluating the most cost-effective package of primary promotion and secondary prevention measures for meeting specific sexual health objectives. Such an evaluation has to take account of interactions between primary and secondary processes and the inherent uncertainties. These include the numbers HIV positive, the number of false positives from the HIV test, and the adequacy of targetting decisions.

Conclusions

From the discussion in this paper three main conclusions can be drawn concerning the rationale for undertaking an economic evaluation of alternative strategies for promoting sexual health.

Firstly, decisions on the use of scarce resources have to be made both between and within health programmes. At one level this involves a choice between the allocation of resources for the prevention of sexually transmitted diseases against using these resources in a different health programme. At a second choice level decisions have to be made on the allocation of resources for the prevention of sexually transmitted diseases to alternative sexual health programmes in order to achieve most benefits. The economic framework described in this paper provides an approach to assist decision makers in this process.

Secondly, the economic framework can be used to enable direct comparison between the alternative options for achieving sexual health objectives. Cost-benefit analysis, cost-effectiveness analysis or cost-utility analysis could be used to examine which of several different preventive programmes appears to provide most value for money. Currently, there is a lack of reliable evidence on the effectiveness of alternative approaches for promoting sexual health. Economists will only be able to play a full role if economic components are built into future evaluative studies. Designing prospective studies to meet economic criteria is not without difficulty. For example, many of the costs and benefits attached to different preventive programmes are intangible and therefore difficult to value. However, the economic framework allows these effects to be identified and explicitly recognised[40].

Thirdly, the choice is not usually between one type of preventive programme and another but between more or less of different programmes. As has been argued earlier in this paper most programmes promoting sexual health are a combination of primary promotion and secondary prevention initiatives. Decision makers, for example, might want to compare the marginal cost-effectiveness of providing additional resources for screening for sexually transmitted diseases against using these additional resources on promoting condom use.

An economic evaluation of sexual health promotion is not a costless activity, but neither is the inefficient use of resources within prevention programmes aimed at serious health problems such as HIV/AIDS. This paper has outlined the practicalities of applying the economic framework and demonstrated the need to incorporate it in the design of prospective and retrospective evaluations of sexual health promotion programmes.

Acknowledgments

Christine Godfrey would like to acknowledge the financial support of the UK Economic and Social Research Council.

References

1. Drummond M F, Davies L M. Topics for economic analysis. *In:* Drummond M F, Davies L M (eds). AIDS: The challenge for economic analysis. Birmingham: Health Services Management Centre in collaboration with the World Health Organisation, 1990.

2. Scitovsky A, Rice D. Estimates of the direct and indirect costs of Acquired Immunodeficiency Syndrome in the US, 1985, 1986 and 1991. Public Health Reports 1987; 102: 5-17.

3. Scitovsky A, Over M. AIDS: Costs of care in the developed and developing world. AIDS 1988; 2 (suppl. 1): 571-81.

4. Rovira J. The economics of AIDS prevention. *In:* Schwefel D, Leidl R, Rovira J, Drummond M F (eds). Economic aspects of AIDS and HIV infection. Berlin: Springer-Verlag, 1990.

5. Williams A. Ethics, clinical freedom and the doctors' role. *In:* Culyer A J, Maynard A K, Posnett J W (eds). Competition in health care: reforming the NHS. London: Macmillan Press, 1990.

6. Godfrey C, Tolley K H. An economic approach to the evaluation of HIV/AIDS health education programmes. Paper presented at the HEA Consultation on the Evaluation of Local HIV/AIDS Health Promotion Initiatives, Bristol Polytechnic, 19 May 1990.

7. Cohen D R, Henderson J B. Health, prevention and economics. Oxford: Oxford University Press, 1988.

8. Birch S, Stoddart G. Promoting healthy behaviour: The importance of economic analysis in policy formulation for AIDS prevention. Health Policy. 1990; **16**: 187-97.

9. O'Brien B. AIDS and subjective risk assessment: perspectives from the decision sciences. *In:* Drummond M F, Davies L M (eds). AIDS: the challenge for economic analysis. Birmingham: Health Services Management Centre in collaboration with the World Health Organisation, 1990.

10. Ross H L. British drink driving policy. Br J Addiction 1988; **83**: 863-65.

11. Zuercher A. The latest AIDS projections for the United States. Health Affairs 1990; **9(2)**: 163-70.

12. Anon. The UK epidemic (item 667). AIDS Newsletter 1989; **4(12)**: 2.

13. Scitovsky A A. Study the cost of HIV-related illnesses: reflections on the moving target. Millbank Quarterly 1989; **67(2)**: 318-44.

14. Anon. The cost of AIDS: a stitch in time. Economist 18 August 1990, 102.

15. Tolley K, Maynard A, Robinson D. HIV-AIDS and social care. Discussion Paper 81. York: Centre for Health Economics, University of York, 1991.

16. Jager J C, Postma M J, van der Bloom D P, et al. Epidemiological models and socio-economic information: methodological aspects of AIDS. HIV scenario analysis. *In:* Schwefel D, Leidl R, Rovira, J, Drummond M F (eds). Economic aspects of AIDS and HIV infection. Berlin: Springer-Verlag, 1990.

17. Mulley A G, Silverstein M D, Dierstag J L. Indications for use of hepatitis B vaccine, based on cost-effectiveness analysis. New Eng J Med 1982; **307**: 644-52.

18. Soloman M Z, DeJong W. Recent sexually transmitted prevention efforts and their implications for AIDS health education. Health Education Quarterly 1986; **13(4)**: 301-16.

19. Sherr L. An evaluation of the UK Government health education campaign on AIDS. Psychology and Health 1987; **1**: 61-72.

20. Ross M W, Rosser B R S. Education and AIDS risks: a review. Health Education Research: Theory and Practice 1989; **4(3)**: 273-84.

21. Coates T J. Strategies for modifying sexual behaviour for primary and secondary prevention of HIV disease. J Consulting and Clinical Psychology 1990; **58(1)**: 57-69.

22. Tolley K, Maynard A. Government funding of HIV-AIDS medical and social care. Discussion Paper 70. York: Centre for Health Economics, University of York, 1990.

23. Mills S, Campbell M J, Waters W E. Public knowledge of AIDS and the DHSS advertisement campaign. Br Med J 1986; **293**: 1089-90.

24. Anon. Advertising and health education messages (item 420). AIDS Newsletter 1990; **5(8)**: 3.

25. Office of Health Economics. HIV and AIDS in the United Kingdom. OHE Briefing No. 23. London: OHE, 1988.

26. Redman S, Spencer E A, Sanson-Fisher R W. The role of mass media in changing health-related behaviour: a critical appraisal of two models. Health Promotion International 1990; **5(1)**: 85-101.

27. Sisk J E, Hewitt M, Metcalf K L. The effectiveness of AIDS education. Health Affairs 1988; **7(5)**: 37-51.

28. Beardshaw V, Hunter D J, Taylor R C R. Local AIDS policies: planning and policy development for health promotion. AIDS Programme Papers 6. London: Health Education Authority, 1990.

29. Department of Health Circular EL(89) P/36. London: Department of Health, February 1989.

30. de Haes W F M, Schuurman J H. Messages, target groups and the effect of an education programme. Hygiene 1985; **4**(3): 19-25.

31. Mohanty K, Bashier Z, Allen J. The role of health education and counselling in the control of HIV. Br J Sexual Medicine 1988; **September**: 299-302.

32. Drummond M F, Ludbrook A, Lowson K, Steele A. Studies in economic appraisal in health care: Volume 2. Oxford: Oxford University Press, 1986.

33. Horsburgh C R, Douglas J M, LaFore F M. Sexually transmitted diseases. J Amer Med Ass 1987; **258**: 814-21.

34. US Preventive Services Task Force. Guide to clinical preventive services. Baltimore: Williams and Wilkins, 1989.

35. Williams K. Screening for syphilis in pregnancy: An assessment of the costs and benefits. Community Medicine 1985; **7**: 37-42.

36. Phin N. Can economics be applied to prenatal screening? Discussion Paper 74. York: Centre for Health Economics, University of York, 1991.

37. Campbell C A. Women and AIDS. Soc Sci Med 1990; **30**(4): 407-16.

38. Anon. Insurance firms retain bias over HIV test. Independent 6 March 1991, 6.

39. Russell L B. Is prevention better than cure? Washington: Brookings Institute, 1986.

40. Godfrey C, Hardman G, Maynard A. Priorities for health promotion: an economic approach. Discussion Paper 59. York: Centre for Health Economics, University of York, 1989.

10

Reflections

Roger Short FRS
Department of Physiology,
Monash University,
Melbourne,
Victoria

Let me begin by thanking the Organisers very much for inviting me to come here all the way from Australia. I have a very special reason for accepting their invitation which will become apparent in a moment. I have been given the title "Reflections", and you will remember what Shakespeare had to say on the subject in Julius Caesar: "And since you know you cannot see yourself so well as by reflection, I, your glass, will modestly discover to yourself that of yourself which you yet know not of". I will take that as my brief.

The reason I leapt at the invitation to come here was that within about ten yards of where I am now standing, I first used a condom for sexual intercourse, thirty-three years ago. I don't think there is any other person here who can claim such a feat. I was living in a little house called "The Cottage", 53 Grange Road, which was the coachman's cottage attached to a big house called Binnbrook, and the brook that ran through the garden was marshy and clogged with brambles and briars. I am sorry that the cottage has been destroyed, but I rented a TV set in those days from a Mr Robinson, and I suppose that it is just desserts that he should have funded the building of this great College which replaced my little cottage. In the process he also cleared the brambles from the Binn brook, which has now become a beautiful feature of Robinson College gardens. So let us try and clear some of the brambles from our thinking about promoting sexual health.

One of my recollections of the fifteen years I spent in Cambridge goes back to the early 1960s. Dr Malcolm Potts, formerly Cambridge University's Proctor responsible for student discipline, and subsequently Medical Director of the International Planned Parenthood Federation, came to give a widely advertised public lecture on Family Planning in which he said that it would be much better for the health of the undergraduate population if the cigarette machines were removed from Junior Common Rooms, and replaced by slot machines selling condoms. I was having dinner at the high table at my College that evening, and the Fellows were deeply shocked by his remarks. "Have you heard what that man Potts has said? He should be run out of town!" I think that is a good example of how you can give the right message to the wrong audience at the wrong time. There is no way you could persuade the Fellows to adopt condoms; they are past it in more than one sense of the word. The lesson that we must learn is that if we are going to do something to improve sexual health, we must target our message to youth, because the young are the ones who are most likely to change their patterns of sexual behaviour; they are also the ones with the highest rate of change of sexual partners, which makes them a particularly vulnerable group.

I would like to introduce the theme of the three Horsemen of the Apocalypse, who left to their own devices will lead mankind to destruction; those three Horsemen are overpopulation, sexually transmitted diseases, and HIV infection and AIDS. Let me talk first about overpopulation.

Population Growth

Every day, a quarter of a million people are added to the population of the earth. Over-population is the transcending problem of our time. We cannot think about reproductive health without relating it first and foremost to containing human population growth. But we now have a new challenge, and that is to try to link contraception to the prevention of sexually transmitted diseases in general and of HIV infection in particular.

Who, in this room, can go back to the place of their birth and find it unchanged? We have brought about staggering changes in the world in a very short space of time. If you would like to walk down Burrell's Lane and then on into Jesus Lane, and enter Jesus College, you will see on the wall a portrait of T R Malthus, a Fellow of that College, who wrote his famous Essay on the Principles of Population in 1798[1]. That is just under two hundred years ago, and at that time there were only 1 billion people on the earth. By 1930, when I was born, numbers had jumped to 2 billion, and to 3 billion by the time I first used a condom. They had reached 4 billion by the 1970's, and 5 billion by the late 1980s. When will it stop?

If we had dropped an atom bomb *every day* since that fateful Monday of August 6th, 1945, when the first atom bomb was dropped on Hiroshima, if we had killed 100,000 people every day since then, we would still not have halted the growth in the human population, although we would have slowed it somewhat. So overpopulation is the most important of the three Horsemen of the Apocalypse; if we cannot rein it in, we face disaster.

Sexually Transmitted Diseases

Then we come to the Second Horseman, sexually transmitted diseases. Let me remind you of the game of conkers. Some of you will have played conkers as children, using the fruit of a horse chestnut tree on a string to alternately smite and be smitten by your opponent's conker. If you smash his conker yours becomes a "one-er", and if you then beat another opponent it becomes a "twoer". But if your twoer cracks someone else's twoer, it becomes a fiver. Playing conkers in a little village school, you may end up with a tenner; but in a big city comprehensive school with a couple of thousand pupils, in one single encounter you might become a one hundred and fiftier. Conker scores increase with population density. Sexually transmitted diseases behave in the same way, since they are cumulative over time. As populations grow in size, sexually transmitted diseases become increasingly prevalent because the number of people playing the game is increased.

Table 1 shows the percentage of women with primary female infertility who are unable to have any children, by country[2]. This is a good indication of the incidence of STDs, which can result in blockage of the Fallopian tubes and hence sterility. In Africa, the prevalence of primary female infertility is very high[3], the record being in Gabon where a staggering 32% of women are unable ever to have a child. In Europe the figures are generally around 6-11%, and most of us have tended to assume that this is perfectly normal and natural, part of Nature's design. But WHO has recently produced some very interesting data from Beijing, showing an incredibly low rate of primary female infertility of only 1.5%. Perhaps this is because China has hitherto had little premarital sex, virtually no divorce or remarriage, very little prostitution, and very little extra-marital sex, and hence there has been very little sexually transmitted disease. If this figure of 1.5% represents the true norm for the incidence of female infertility, then the higher levels in Europe probably reflect quite a high incidence of sexually transmitted disease. The very high figure for Gabon appears to be explained by the fact that, in that country, young girls start intercourse at the age of 12, two years before their periods start, and their first acts of intercourse are with older men[4]. If you increase the age differential between the partners, you greatly increase the chances of the younger partner becoming infected with sexually transmitted diseases, since the older partner unknowingly transmits the accumulated venereal experiences of a lifetime: unknowingly, because many sexually transmitted diseases are asymptomatic.

So what can we do about reducing the incidence of sexually transmitted diseases? In Britain, we refurbish a beautiful old country house just outside Cambridge, Bourne Hall, and turn it into an *in vitro* fertilization clinic, and we make test tube babies available on the National Health Service, at a cost of thousands of pounds per cycle of treatment. But condoms are not available from general practitioners under the National Health Service. Haven't we got our priorities hopelessly wrong? An ounce of prevention is infinitely preferable to a few thousand pounds of cure.

On September 22, 1497 the Town Council of Edinburgh held an emergency meeting to discuss the sudden appearance of a new contagious Distemper, supposed to be venereal, called the Grandgore[5]. It had arrived in Edinburgh in the aftermath of the raising of the Siege of Naples in 1495, and this disease, later to be called syphilis, was spread all over Europe by the disbanded mercenary army of King Charles VIII of France. He had failed to capture Naples because his forces were decimated by syphilis; it seems likely that the infection had come from some of Christopher Columbus's crew, who had returned from the Caribbean on March 15, 1493, bringing the infection with them, and had subsequently enlisted with Gonzalo de Cordoba who joined forces with King Charles in mounting the Siege of Naples[6].

The Scots decided that in order to prevent the spread of this dreaded new disease, all infected individuals were to be banished to the Island of Inchcolme in the Firth of Forth, which is a pretty bare, barren, inhospitable island. Anyone who was subsequently found to be infected and still at large in the city "Salle be brynt on the cheik with the marking irne that thai may be kennit in tym to cum"[5]. So stigmatisation because of sexually transmitted disease has a very long history. But at least with syphilis there were outward and visible signs that a person was infected, and this made it possible to contain spread. From a public health point of view it is far more difficult to deal with asymptomatic venereal infections in which the individual remains infectious to others. Screening is not a viable option, particularly when there is no cure on offer.

Table 1: Percentage of women unable to have any children

Region	Country	Percentage
Africa	Cameroon	15
	Central African Republic	17
	Congo	21
	Gabon	32
	Ivory Coast	10
	Tanzania	10
	Zaire	21
	Zambia	14
Asia	Bangladesh	4
	China	1.5
	Indonesia	7
	Thailand	2
Americas	Mexico	3
	USA	9
Europe	Belgium	7
	Denmark	6
	France	6
	Spain	4
	Sweden	11
	UK	6

Source: Ref 2.

It was syphilis that led Gabriel Fallopio in 1564 to develop the condom. In his book *De Morbo Gallico* he says the following:

> "As often as a man has intercourse, he should (if possible) wash the genitals, or wipe them with a cloth; afterward he should use a small linen cloth made to fit the glans, and draw forward the prepuce over the glans; if he can do so, it is well to moisten it with saliva or with a lotion; however, it does not matter .... I tried the experiment on eleven hundred men, and I call immortal God to witness that not one of them was infected".[7]

We have never thought of using a condom for *post-coital* STD prevention, and although it would only protect the man and not the woman, perhaps we should develop Fallopius' ideas further. A suitably medicated cap placed over the glans after intercourse might be the ideal way of delivering bactericidal or virucidal drugs to the site at which organisms are most likely to enter the male reproductive tract, namely the urethral meatus.

HIV and AIDS

Just as syphilis arrived at the end of the 15th century and spread terror throughout Europe, so today at the end of the 20th century we are suddenly faced with another new sexually transmitted disease, HIV infection. WHO estimates that by June 1990 there were somewhere between 8-10 million HIV positive people, and it projects a cumulative total of 40 million HIV infections by the year 2000.

Where did this infection come from? It seems likely that it came from chimpanzees, for there has recently been a report of a wild chimpanzee in Gabon with HIV antibodies from which a virus was isolated which, on sequencing, was virtually indistinguishable from HIV1[8]. So how did this virus jump from chimpanzees into humans? Not by bestiality, which is highly unlikely, but much more simply. It would only need a hunter to cut his hand when skinning an infected animal for him to be infected.

We can speculate that HIV may have been jumping from chimpanzees into humans for thousands of years. At low human population densities in Africa's tropical rainforests, the home of the chimpanzee, the chances of infected humans spreading the disease beyond their immediate family would be almost zero. But as human numbers have built up around chimpanzee habitats, and as tracks and roads have begun to penetrate the dwindling forests, the

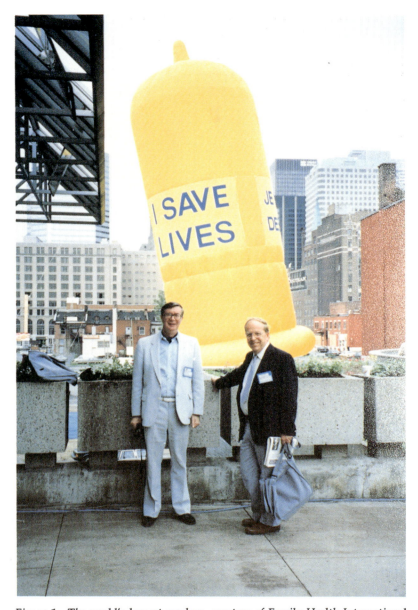

Figure 1: *The world's largest condom, courtesy of Family Health International.*

chances of spread within the human population have increased. Perhaps one successful hunter bought a bicycle, which enabled him to cycle into the nearest village of an evening, and have sex with a girl who subsequently had sex with a lorry driver, thereby putting a match to the kindling and initiating the HIV pandemic.

A Solution

So how can we rein in these three horsemen of the Apocalypse? The Alma Ata Declaration of 1978 promised "Health for all by the year 2000", and this has become the slogan of WHO. Doesn't it have a hollow ring about it? The concept is hopelessly flawed in the aftermath of HIV. I would suggest that this conference might counter with the Cambridge Question: "Health for *whom* by the year 2000?" It certainly will not be health for all. Those who are denied health are the ones to whom we should target our preventative strategies.

Table 2: Percentage of couples using contraceptives who choose the condom

Region	Country	Year	% condom use
Africa	Burundi	1987	0
	Cameroon	1978	0
	Ghana	1980	1
	Ivory Coast	1981	0
	Kenya	1984	0
	Rwanda	1983	0
Americas	Brazil	1986	2
	Canada	1984	8
	Dominican Republic	1986	1
	Haiti	1983	1
	Mexico	1987	2
	Trinidad and Tobago	1987	12
	USA	1982	10
Asia and Pacific	China	1985	2
	India	1982	5
	Japan	1983	45
	New Zealand	1976	8
	Singapore	1983	24
	Thailand	1987	1
Europe	Denmark	1981	25
	Finland	1977	32
	France	1978	6
	W Germany	1985	6
	Italy	1979	13
	The Netherlands	1985	7
	Spain	1985	12
	Sweden	1981	25
	Switzerland	1980	8
	UK	1983	17

Source: Ref 9.

How can we keep population growth, sexually transmitted diseases and HIV infection all at bay? Aside from celibacy or lifelong mutual monogamy, neither of which comes easily to a polygamous primate like ourselves, we have only one true preventative, and that is a condom. How can we increase condom acceptability?

If we look at the percentage of couples using contraception who choose the condom (Table 2)[9], we see that in Europe, Finland, Sweden and Denmark are setting an example, so we should be listening to them. But when we look at the rest of the world, Africa has user rates of between 0 and 1%. How can we deploy the condom in such countries to have a meaningful impact? In the Americas, Trinidad and Tobago and the USA have some condom use but in other countries there is very little. In Asia and the Pacific, the shining example is Japan with 45% condom use. Surely we can learn from the Japanese how to make condoms more acceptable? We must target youth, and our challenge is to get condoms into the classroom. The condom must become the contraceptive of first choice for all young people starting sexual activity, because it is the only thing that will prevent unwanted pregnancies, STDs that result in infertility, and HIV infection that results in death.

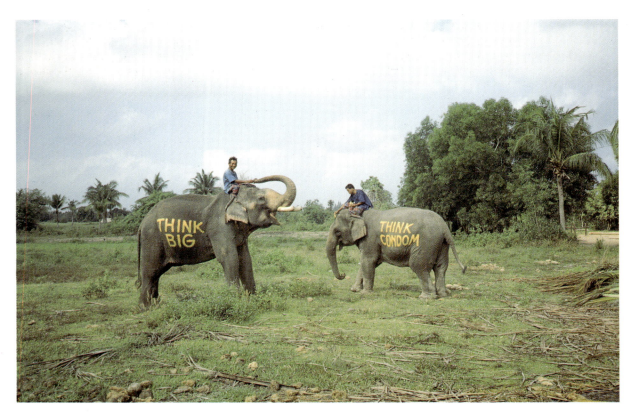

Figure 2: A jumbo condom promotion in Thailand.

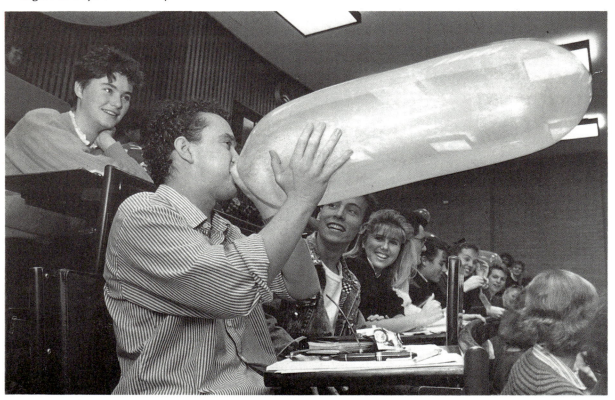

Figure 3: An essential part of medical school training?   *See Ref 10.*

How might we change attitudes to condoms? Malcolm Potts and I had Family Health International build the world's largest condom. It is 125ft tall and we flew it at Montreal at the International AIDS conference in 1989 with the logo "I save lives; je sauve la vie" (Figure 1). It was interesting to see the public reaction, which was really quite favourable. We then entered it for the International Hot Air Balloon Festival in Albuquerque, New Mexico, where it was banned as obscene. It was even banned in Raleigh, North Carolina, Family Health International's home town.

Would the Health Education Authority dare to fly that condom in Britain? It would be nice to see it floating in Britain's friendly skies, because it is an excellent barometer of public opinion. There are other ways of promoting condoms. The elephant is a symbol of sagacity throughout Asia, and also a very good billboard. We have therefore used Thai elephants for condom promotion (Figure 2).

WHO is a bit like an elephant; it is very impressive, expensive to keep, and ponderously slow, but it produces loud noises from both ends that make people listen, and it is very wise. But I've heard remarkably little from either the Geneva or the Copenhagen ends of WHO about condoms. Could you please trumpet a little louder in future, because we need the authority of WHO in a global campaign to promote condoms? But each of us can also do some promotion. Figure 3 shows a class of medical students at Monash University all blowing up condoms[10], and everyone is laughing. I don't think any doctor ought to be allowed to qualify until he has come face to face with a condom and blown it up until it bursts. It is a remarkably effective way of desensitizing you to condoms for life. We subsequently use our desensitised students to give safe sex instruction to all Monash undergraduates when they first enter the University, and this peer group educational exercise appears to be remarkably successful.

So in conclusion, if we look around this room, we see an interesting assortment of people, of different religions, creeds, colours, beliefs and behaviours, but we are all here because we are united in one thing: to try and rein in those three Horsemen of the Apocalypse who will otherwise lead us to destruction. And until we have something better, the condom is all that we have to deploy. Let's make full use of it.

Spencer Hagard: Thank you very much indeed, especially for the hot air challenge which I'm going to accept on behalf of the HEA. We will try and get this condom flying above Britain's skies this summer. We will do our best. A couple of points for discussion please?

Maria Paalman: Could you comment on the joint use of the contraceptive pill and the condom because in The Netherlands, as you well know, we have a very low teenage pregnancy rate. The Family Planning Association has always said that it is due to a low rate of condom use for contraception, with very high use of the pill among young women. Promoting condoms is not done in The Netherlands at this moment to prevent pregnancy. So the message given is "Use a pill to not get pregnant, use a condom to not get sick". Could you comment on that?

Roger Short: Of course it is always better to wear a belt and braces, because then your trousers really won't fall down. My worry about promoting condoms plus the pill is, how many of us in this room are actually wearing a belt and braces? And if he knows she is on the pill, can she still persuade him to use a condom? I think we can take comfort from Sweden where they have had a very successful condom promotion campaign and pill use has declined markedly. The incidence of gonorrhoea has declined abruptly since 1975, but there has been only a very slight increase in the incidence of teenage pregnancies. One of the recommendations of the condom working group is the need for more information about condom use-effectiveness and method-effectiveness for pregnancy prevention. The Swedish experience is encouraging and I think that we are probably on fairly safe grounds in promoting condoms on their own as a contraceptive, but I do have some concern, and I'm very glad you asked me that question.

References

1. Malthus T R. Essay on the principle of population as it affects the future improvement of society. 1798.

2. Farley T M M, Belsey E M. The prevalence and ætiology of infertility. Int Union for the Scientific Study of Population, African Population Conference, Dakar Senegal 1988; **1**: 2.1.15-2.1.30.

3. Collet M, Reniers J, Frost E, Gass R, Yvert F, Leclerc A, Roth-Meyer C, Ivanoff B, Meheus A. Infertility in Central Africa: infection is the cause. Int J Gynecol Obstet 1988; **26**: 423-428.

4. Mavoungou D, Frost E, Collet M, Gass R, Leclerc A, Peeters M. Sexuality, puberty and sexually transmitted diseases (STD in young African girls in Gabon. *In:* Teoh E-S, Ratnam S S, Seng K M (eds). Advances in fertility and sterility. Vol 5, Endometriosis. Proc 12th World Congr on Fertil Steril, Singapore. New Jersey: Parthenon Publishing, 1986, 137-139.

5. Part of a letter from Mr Macky, Professor of History, to Mr MacLaurin, Professor of Mathematics in the University of Edinburgh, and by him communicated to the President of the Royal Society; being an extract from the books of the Town Council of Edinburgh, relating to a disease there, supposed to be venereal, in the year 1497. Phil Trans Roy Soc 1743; **42**: 420-421.

6. Cartwright F F. Disease and history. New York: Thomas Cromwell C, 1972, 58-59.

7. Hines N E. Medical history of contraception. New York: Gamut, 1963, 190.

8. Huet T, Cheynier R, Meyerhaus A, Roelants G, Wain-Hobson S. Genetic organisation of a chimpanzee lentivirus related to HIV-1. Nature 1990; **345**: 356-358.

9. Mauldin W P, Segal S J. Prevalence of contraceptive use: trends and issues. Studies in Family Planning 1988; **19**: 335-353.

10. Short R V. Teaching AIDS. IPPF Medical Bulletin 1989; **23(3)**: 1-4.

11

AIDS/HIV and Sexual Health in Relation to the General Population

Report by Kaye Wellings (chairperson of working group), Academic Department of Public Health, St Mary's Hospital Medical School, London

Other working group members were:

Jo Adams	*UK*
Nikolai Chaika	*USSR*
Gauden Galea	*Malta*
Enrique García Huete	*Spain*
Alan Glanz	*UK*
James Halloran	*UK*
Margaret Jay	*UK*
Crista Jebelean	*Romania*
Odd Einar Johansen	*Norway*
Lilian Kolker	*The Netherlands*
Zdeněk Kučera	*Czechoslovakia*
Susan Perl	*UK*
Kate Pocock	*UK*
Donald Reid	*UK*
Roger Tyrrell	*UK*
Simon Sandberg	*UK*
Zofia Słońska	*WHO/Poland*

What Do We Mean by the Term "General Population"?

An important task preliminary to any discussion of sexual health education in relation to the *general population* is to provide an operational definition of the term. All too often, the "general population" is conceived of as the residual mass of people which is left when so called high risk groups are taken out. As such it tends to be equated with a non-drug using, heterosexual population, and is assumed to be homogeneous, finite and discrete.

In practice of course, people do not assemble themselves in such neat pigeon-holes. They move in and out of categories of "at-riskness" through different stages and phases of life, with place and time, as their situations change. The average heterosexual youngster in a village in Gloucestershire, in the Basque or in Jutland may be at relatively low risk at home, but on vacation the risk may increase. Similarly , sexual relationships tend to be temporally dynamic. Couples may be at low risk because they are currently monogamous, but their status will change rapidly should the relationship break down and they may find themselves back at the stage of changing partners. In addition, people constantly rediscover their sexual orientation. Old audiences are thus replaced by new ones as people mature into behaviours or move from one life stage to another.

Further, people cannot be relied upon to identify as members of particular groups on the strength of shared behaviour patterns (and indeed may be reluctant to do so where such behaviours are socially stigmatised) and so cannot be targeted directly and specifically, but only at the aggregate level. Additionally, HIV may be acquired as a consequence of one risk behaviour, but passed on as a result of another, so that there is little to be gained from addressing particular behaviours exclusively.

A preferable way of looking at the general population then seems to be in terms of *communicational strategy* rather than *risk group*. The communicational strategy linked with the general population will by definition be a broad spectrum approach, rather than the targetted approach, whether at the level of mass media, school education or community level education.

Any messages need to take account of the heterogeneous nature of such a population. We are concerned in this group with people whose behaviour may put them at risk but who may not see themselves as part of a 'high risk group'. But we are also concerned with people who are at very little risk. Every effort needs to be made to avoid frightening people unnecessarily. AIDS is everybody's problem, but not a problem of the same order of magnitude for everyone.

Although there may not be a need for everyone to change their behaviour, there may be a need for everyone to acquire knowledge of, and appropriate attitudes towards, sexual health. Mobilising the whole population allows open and free discussion which will benefit minorities. There is little point in encouraging young people in the school setting to speak more freely and openly about sexuality if on their return home they find the discourse closes up on them. And there is little point in encouraging those at risk to be open about their practices if in doing so they risk being met by public opprobrium.

An appropriate medium: mass media vs community level approaches

The broad spectrum approach is equated in the minds of many with the use of the mass media, and indeed the past decade has seen the use of this communicational means on a scale unprecedented in health education. Major achievements and advances have been made. In most European countries, at least those in which evaluative data has been collected, awareness of, and information about, HIV and AIDS is perhaps higher than for almost any other disease. In addition, great progress has been made in shifting some of the old shibboleths – the taboo on condom advertising, on sexual explicitness, etc.

Yet however effective use of the mass media has been, in terms of raising awareness and transmitting information, the European experience points time and again to the shortcomings of this approach in terms of achieving the requisite changes in behaviour. From Spain we hear of the failure of the mass media to reach prostitutes in Catalonia; from the UK there is the example of lack of observable change in young people, and so on. We now seem to have reached a ceiling in terms of what can be achieved by this means.

The most effective way of prompting the motivation necessary for behaviour change would seem to be by face-to-face communication at local or community level, where messages can be tailored to the specific needs of individuals and need not be trimmed to take account of official and statutory sensitivities.

Yet the recognition that mass media campaigns may not be effective in changing behaviour should not prompt us to abandon our efforts in this direction. There is general agreement that mass media provides support for and validation of interventions at community level. Regular reinforcing messages via the mass media and central agencies of communication are necessary to those working with high risk behaviour as well as legitimising the position of AIDS on the social and political agenda.

Thus in relation to the possible shift towards working with specific target audiences and community level approaches, this group felt that this could only take place hand in hand with the continuation of broad spectrum programmes. The media can create contexts of acceptability and agenda setting which are essential for those working at grass root level. A strong need emerges for a national voice, to maintain global campaigns aimed at the general population in order to reinforce and provide credibility to community activities, particularly initiatives related to the general public.

Thus national and community approaches co-exist symbiotically. The relationship between mass media and more personal communication is mutually beneficial in the sense that issues are flagged up at national level and acted on at local level. Personal communication depends on AIDS being recognised officially as a continuing issue, just as the broad spectrum approach depends on messages being picked up and worked on through more interpersonal communication. In order for this symbiosis to be exploited, a strong link is needed between national campaigns and community work, to ensure continuity and harmony between the two.

An appropriate message

A tempting strategy during European level discussions is to compile an inventory of messages which can be used in the fight against AIDS. There are, however, major problems to be faced in agreeing on messages of universal value. In general, messages are determined by campaign aims and objectives. The two fundamental aims of interventions in relation to HIV/AIDS are firstly, to reduce the risk of infection by encouraging appropriate behaviour and, secondly, to create a favourable social context within which prevention activities and the care and treatment of those affected can be carried out. The strength with this second objective is stated in campaigns in different countries varies from the weakly phrased "reducing social disruption" to the more explicitly stated "promoting solidarity" or "creating a favourable environment".

There is now a gradual recognition that public education efforts to date have been marked by an over-reliance on individual behaviour change and an insufficient emphasis on creating a favourable social context. As the numbers of those affected increase, this will be an increasingly important focus of attention. In this area, broad spectrum approaches to AIDS/HIV prevention can make a major contribution. A start can be made at European level by disseminating messages of solidarity campaigns – for example, from The Netherlands *"No one got HIV from giving a little understanding"*; from Norway *"Human care is not contagious"*; and from France, *"Le SIDA chacun de nous peut le rencontrer"* – in countries in which such an approach has not yet been tackled.

More is likely to be achieved in this respect, however, by exchange of information relating to efforts addressed at opinion formers, including the unpaid-for media. This may be less costly than efforts directed at the general public, but may require considerably more resourcefulness and ingenuity. A helpful bishop, a sympathetic editorial, a concerned comment from a politician cannot be paid for, but are worth their weight in gold, and every effort needs to be made to exploit such opportunities nationally and to share the experience internationally.

Specific Issues

A number of issues feature more prominently in a discussion of HIV/AIDS public education addressed to the general population than they do in discussions about efforts relating to particular target groups: the difficulty of sustaining interest and maintaining a place for HIV/AIDS on the public agenda; and the problem of handling sensitive material in the public domain. Discussion centering on the general population constantly returns to these themes.

Sustainability

Ten years into the AIDS epidemic, the worst possible scenarios predicted for widespread spread of HIV into the general population have fortunately not been realised in most European countries. Nevertheless, as has always been recognised, the threat of HIV infection remains an intractable problem, requiring long term vigilance. We are now facing problems of maintaining a constant presence for HIV/AIDS in public education campaigns, at the same time as attempting to 'normalize' the disease, moving away from a concept of acute crisis to one of a chronic public health problem.

One identifiable difficulty is that sustainability is often in opposition to authenticity. Exaggerating the level of risk will destroy credibility, whilst honestly stating it may not be sufficient to motivate people. Overstating the case, as in the heavily fear-dominated early campaigns in the UK and in Australia, for example, has resulted in interventions which are difficult to follow up, and confusing for the public when the most pessimistic predictions are clearly not observable.

The problem is compounded by the threat of shrinking resources. At present relatively lavish budgets are still dedicated to AIDS/HIV preventive activities, and there is strong government approval for preventive work, but there is no guarantee that this situation will continue, and indeed there are already signs of diminishing and declining interest at some levels. There is therefore a need to have structures in place now, in anticipation of and preparation for possible "years of famine" in the future.

In such circumstances the need to avoid so-called "bolt-on" interventions – ad hoc, unco-ordinated and lacking continuity – and instead to discover and implement sustainable approaches, is paramount. A major problem of AIDS/HIV public education in some countries has been its disjointed and uneven pace. Interventions need to be paced to avoid short, intermittent and apparently unconnected bursts of publicity. Public education campaigns in some countries have achieved considerable success in keeping AIDS and HIV on the public agenda by this means and have helped guard against the "here today gone tomorrow" spirit which seems to be generated by high profile hyper-activity followed by periods of relative inactivity.

One means by which this has been achieved has been by incorporating a synergistic element into the campaign format by employing a continuing theme, logo, motif or slogan – the ubiquitous condom shape in Switzerland, as the moon over Geneva, the sun on holiday, the "O" of tonight and OK; the sound of a whistle in Denmark marking every TV ad; the *"Si Da, No Da"* slogan in Spain – have all helped continuity and economy of message. Others have achieved sustainability by pacing interventions and ensuring a regular and controlled level of information. In The Netherlands, the endline of the most recent campaign, *"AIDS is still with us"* reminds people of the continuing need for care.

The problem of sustainability is not, of course, applicable as yet to Eastern Europe. There, AIDS public education is just beginning. Not only is the duration of the AIDS epidemic shorter in these countries, but the lack of established health promotion structures has delayed response to it in terms of public education. Add to this an unstable economic and political situation, and the lack of networks to use for the purpose, and it is not surprising that AIDS initiatives have been slow to get off the ground.

Recent experience in these countries cautions against the instant transfer of tried and tested strategies from the West, and a parallel respect for the cultural, political and economic national constraints. Campaigns are necessarily to some extent culturally specific, so that what works in one country or with one group may not in another. In many Eastern European countries a biomedical approach to public health is dominant so that screening and testing have been seen as more appropriate interventions than information, education and communication. The National AIDS Federations in Hungary and Bulgaria, for example, have invested major efforts in mandatory screening with special emphasis on groups such as travellers, prostitutes, etc.

The move in these countries, from biomedical approaches to prevention towards a greater reliance on health promotion, is slow. Where health issues are very medicalised, the population becomes passive and expects to be served by doctors and not to have to take control over their own destiny. An established dependence on medical approaches to stopping the spread of disease is, as a consequence, problematic for health promotion.

Sensitivity

Sensitivity in public education is identified as a more substantial issue in the context of activities targetted at the general population than to those directed to smaller target groups. Activities at the level of general public health education are high-profile and visibility is unavoidable. Generally, because of the scale of the exercise and the costs involved, governmental involvement in campaigns is inevitable, which brings further problems in terms of what is possible with regard to sexual explicitness and openness. Additionally, and increasingly problematically, as the threat of a large scale epidemic of HIV and AIDS in the general population recedes in many European countries, so does enthusiasm for espousing the more radical and controversial measures.

The difficulty of handling more sensitive health educational material in relation to sexual health in general, and HIV and AIDS in particular, is well illustrated by reference to the kinds of messages being transmitted. Whilst some, for example, "restrict numbers of partners/adopt monogamy" clearly underpin the moral code, others, for example, "use a condom during sex with someone you are not sure of" might be seen by some to undermine it. Yet the most effective health education messages, as is well established, offer a choice of realisable messages to the public. These are optimally presented in terms of a hierarchy of fail-safe messages; in the case of messages relating to drug use, the list would run:

- Don't use drugs at all;
- If you can't avoid using drugs, don't inject them;
- If you must inject for the present, don't share needles;
- If you ever share needles, make sure you sterilise them first.

In general the further down the hierarchy the message is to be found, the greater its potential credibility with target groups but the more sensitive it is in political terms, and the more difficulties might be encountered in finding acceptance at the official level. Conversely, the higher the message in the hierarchy the less likely it is that it will earn the trust and confidence of the target group, but the more likely it is to gain political acceptance.

Whilst virtually no European country has escaped some political difficulty in transmitting the condom message, varying degrees of success have been achieved in circumventing the sources of opposition. Some countries have done unexpectedly well in this respect. In Spain for example, a country whose Catholic tradition might have been expected to militate against the frank and explicit presentation of pragmatic messages to use condoms, major progress has been made in deflecting opposition through the use of cartoon characters depicting safe and unsafe sex. In Norway, too, the use of humour has helped ease the passage of some of the more explicit campaign components.

The HIV/AIDS epidemic has opened doors which no one thought possible. In the UK for example, the British Broadcasting Corporation refused to screen the Grand Prix in 1985 because Durex sponsored one car, and TV advertising of condoms was forbidden. Yet only two years later, in July 1987, this ban was lifted and the first TV condom commercial was screened.

Countries can clearly learn from one another but must always be aware of the cultural, social and political constraints in each. Local campaigns may avoid causing offence where similar ones at central level would run into difficulties. Health educators in Western Europe often forget that progress in the West in changing public attitudes has been gradual and incremental rather than radical and revolutionary, and it may be necessary for countries in the East to follow this process.

Experience in this respect again cautions against the belief that materials used in the West transport easily or automatically to the East. Orthodox Catholics oppose most of the interventions in Poland and it is impossible to use the mass media in relation to condom messages. A gay leaflet for gay men on safer sex translated from the French original was seen as dangerous and as encouraging homosexuality. In Romania, for example, a visitor from The Netherlands brought text on the use of condoms for use with factory workers, but the translator refused to translate the most explicit sections. In that country anyway, the quality of condoms produced is too poor for their promotion. A problem is also encountered in relation to the use of methadone in Poland where it is seen as unethical to exchange one drug for another.

In Western European countries again, the assumption is often made that more sensitive work can be handled by NGOs, so as to relieve the government of embarrassment and harmful controversy. But we must be careful not to take for granted that all countries are well provided with such an infrastructure. Czechoslovakia, for example, is lacking in this respect. There, institutions are highly medicalised. Alternatetively, there may be an established framework of non-governmental organisation but the problem lies in how to use it.

Nevertheless, experiences in coping with unfavourable climates in one country may be extremely valuable to another. Certainly health educators in different European countries can learn from one another, and should do so increasingly if possibly diminishing resources are to be preserved. Every effort should be made to exchange information about successes and failures. Some of the mistakes made in earlier campaigns in the West are in danger of being repeated; for example, in Czechoslovakia, campaigners are using high levels of fear and there is little or no promotion of sexual enjoyment.

Broadening the Remit of HIV/AIDS to Sexual Health

Mooting this idea within the general population group met with less enthusiasm than might have been expected. The move both nationally and internationally (in organisations like WHO, the IPPF, the UK HEA etc.), etc. is increasingly towards the integration of HIV and AIDS with other sexual health education. The advantages of such a move are clear. Broadening the remit could help solve the problems relating to perception of risk. Whilst the negative utility attached to the outcome of HIV infection is fairly devastating, the actual probabilities are small in scale so that it is difficult to persuade people to change their behaviour because of the low odds of being affected. Other STDs may be less serious in terms of morbidity and certainly mortality, but are more common, which makes it easier to appeal to people's logic.

Furthermore, the settings of STD clinics, family planning clinics, etc. are useful ones for disseminating messages about sexual health, particularly since in these contexts people present voluntarily with a sexually related problem or health condition and therefore expect relevant advice. It then becomes a relatively easy task to broaden that advice to other aspects of sexual health.

Then again, HIV/AIDS has pushed things forward in many countries in terms of sexual health education, and it would be a mistake not to seize opportunities which now present themselves. In the past, opportunities to get across messages about sexual health have been missed because we have neglected sex education. HIV/AIDS presents an opportunity to remedy this in the wider context of sexually transmitted diseases, psychosexual issues, fertility and infertility, etc.

At the same time, however, a note of caution must be introduced in this context. Issues around healthy sexuality are not simply to do with the avoidance of disease. One consequence of the domination of the sexual health agenda by HIV is that young people particularly may see all STDs as fatal, and sexual activity as life-threatening rather than life-enhancing. Sexually transmitted diseases are still deeply embarrassing, having connotations of sexual profligacy, inconstancy and incontinence. We need to ensure that we do not talk about pathological aspects of sexuality to the exclusion of pleasure. Further, risk reduction practices may not be the same for each aspect of sexual health. For example, a woman attempting to avoid pregnancy may not choose condom use as the most effective means of doing so.

Broadening HIV/AIDS programmes to incorporate not just other STDs, but also issues relating to fertility has therefore advantages and disadvantages. As interest in HIV/AIDS wanes, it clearly makes sense to widen the health issue. On the other hand, in so doing, we must guard against the risk of mixing messages and confusing the public.

Evaluation

In the face of such an urgent health problem as AIDS, emerging as precipitately as it did, the need for evaluation at all is a valid topic for discussion. Almost a decade ago, AIDS appeared on the public health scene with no warning and with little or no time to set up necessary research procedures. Reports now come from Eastern Europe that there has been no time to properly organise campaigns themselves, particularly in the context of internal turmoil where communications are difficult, let alone evaluations.

Certainly there are, in Europe, examples of "conviction campaigns" which appear to have been very successful. The Norwegian campaigns, for example, were founded on the belief that the accumulated wisdom of the health educators involved was sufficient to guide the interventions, and that evaluation was an unnecessary, costly and time-consuming luxury. Ask people what is needed in campaigns, said those who executed the campaigns, and they will very probably say they want to see hospital beds filled with people with AIDS, but this we know from sound and academically tested academic principles to be misguided.

Yet where resources are limited, and campaigns have a high political profile, it is important to make efforts to determine which initiatives are most efficacious. The conclusion of the group was not that evaluation should not be carried out at all, but that it should be carried out differently and with improvements. To this end, an attempt was made to identify flaws in existing evaluations, and ways in which they might be eradicated.

Effectiveness can only relate to declared aims and objectives. Following directly from the operational goals, the central focus of evaluative efforts in relation to the general population to date has been the individual, rather than the social context. In addition, perhaps because of the dominant epidemiological and medical discourse, the focus has been on quantitative pseudo-scientific methods rather than qualitative methods. And since it is mass media approaches which are so cost intensive, evaluative efforts have tended to be concentrated in this area, to the neglect of community approaches.

It is in respect of these three areas of weakness that improvements are recommended. Efforts are urged to seek more effective methods of assessing the extent and nature of changes in the social context, through the use of mass media studies, official discourse analysis, the examination of documentary sources, etc. It is important to evaluate all media campaigns aimed at the general public thoroughly and include a systematic assessment of effects on opinion formers, etc.

Recognising the limited role of the mass media, we must look at this agency in the context of the broader social structure. The mass media can only work through nexus of institutions in society. Information is not communication. The focus must be on the communicational process and not simply assimilation of official messages, so that we need to look at concepts such as access, reception, etc. What are the barriers to internalisation of messages? What are the sources of discord and discontinuity, contradiction and confusion?

Accepting that evaluation has the political function of ratifying and legitimating efforts made, we must nevertheless build into our evaluation the possibility of revealing that we might have got it wrong. We need to allow ourselves to make mistakes and must learn to be confident enough to admit this if others are to learn from our experience. AIDS education permits of no one "magic button" or universal "quick fix"; all campaign components will be culturally and subculturally relative.

In addition, methods need to be devised and developed to assess the unintended effects of campaigns – often very important. Paid for advertising often leads to unpaid for publicity, and our current evaluative tools do not always take this into account. For example, HIV has helped people to talk about sexuality, which must be seen as positive in the context of prevention.

To date, evaluation of community approaches has been neglected. Examples of good practice in this area need to be collected and disseminated. Evaluation techniques in all areas need to be diversified and innovative methods and alternatives to traditional practice considered.

Finally, we must consider alternatives to the quantitative methods of research currently dominating evaluation. The stock-in-trade of evaluation research has been the knowledge attitude and behaviour (KAB) survey, which suffers from the well-documented defects of only measuring change at the individual level, and not at that of the social context. And relying as it does on reported as opposed to observed behaviour, with attendant susceptibility to the desirability response, it presents obvious problems of reliability and validity. If we want better to understand people's motivation in acting in particular ways, and the meaning behaviours have for individuals; if we want to understand and explain and not merely to observe and describe, then an appropriate mix of in-depth qualitative as well as quantitaive techniques need to be employed.

Recommendations

- Resources should be made available for exchange between those working in the field of AIDS/HIV prevention, both in relation to the experience of setting up public education campaigns, and their evaluation. To this end, a co-ordinating centre without copyright should be set up, and materials collected in a location accessible to all. Exchange between Western and Eastern countries, with special attention to building informational networks, should be established with some urgency.

- Centralised global and national campaigns addressed to the general population should be maintained alongside local initiatives, in order to reinforce, legitimate and provide credibility to community activities. All avenues of communication should be used ranging from mass media campaigns to face-to-face communication. Repetition of campaign components will be necessary.

- Messages at the mass media level should be unambiguous and simple, with more complicated messages transmitted at local level and community level.

- Messages need to be incorporated in broad educational messages about healthy sexuality, though this should be in a flexible and non-doctrinaire manner. The distinguishing character of health promotion messages relating to specific health issues needs to be borne in mind at all times.

- Methods of evaluation appropriate to evaluation of changes wrought in the social context should be explored and developed, avoiding a narrow reliance on KABP surveys. Techniques for evaluation should be diversified, utilising an optimal mix of qualitative and quantitative techniques.

- Every country should formulate "lessons for others" as by-product of successes and failures.

- All countries must strengthen the infrastructure for school health education and ensure an appropriate focus on decision-making skills, communication and assertiveness skills.

12

Young People, Sexual Health and HIV/AIDS

Report by Peter Aggleton (author of background paper), Director, Health and Education Research Unit, Goldsmiths' College, University of London, and Peter Dankmeijer (chairperson) Dutch Centre for Health Education and Health Promotion, Utrecht

Other members of the group were:

Janka Beniaková	*Czechoslovakia*
Béla Buda	*Hungary*
John Catford	*UK*
Hannah Cinamon	*UK*
Marina Davoli	*Italy*
Marianna Diomidis	*Greece*
Carmen Fearne	*Malta*
Éva Fébó	*Hungary*
James Hodgkinson	*UK*
Susan Kippax	*Australia*
Merete Lindholm	*Denmark*
Linda Mentens	*Belgium*
Pilar Nájera	*Spain*
Christiana Nöstlinger	*Austria*
Danielle Piette	*Belgium*
Ljudmilla Prììmägi	*Estonia*
Panayot Randev	*Bulgaria*
Christina Rogala	*Sweden*
Manuela Santos Pardal	*Portugal*
Valerie Will	*UK*

Introduction

Young people are frequently identified as a key audience for HIV/AIDS health promotion. In part, this is understandable, given the fact that there are high rates of unintended teenage pregnancy in some countries[1,2,3], and that in others the reported incidence of sexually transmitted diseases (STDs) is highest amongst young people[4]. There is also evidence that many young people become sexually experienced at an earlier age than was the case some years ago[1]. Adolescent health was incorporated into the 8th General Programme of Work of the World Health Organisation which set the following objectives for work in this area:

1. Lower rates of exposure to and contraction of STDs;

2. Greater availability of services to promote young people's reproductive health;

3. A decreased incidence of pregnancy before maturity[5].

While HIV disease may create new challenges for health education and health promotion, its advent provides a useful stimulus to intersectoral work harnessing the energy, insight and resourcefulness of young people themselves. Here we will reflect on some of the options available, having first examined the evidence relating to the risks young people face. We will begin by briefly reviewing aspects of the current epidemiology of HIV and AIDS amongst young people in Europe. Having done this, we will critically evaluate a number of taken-for-granted assumptions about young people and their health promotion needs. Finally, we will discuss some priorities for HIV/AIDS health education and health promotion with young people and amongst those adults with whom they come into contact.

European Epidemiology

14,090 people had been diagnosed as HIV antibody positive by the end of June 1990 in the United Kingdom. Of these, 3,122 (22%) were under the age of 25. By this same point, 3,319 people had been diagnosed with AIDS, of whom 228 (7%) were under the age of 25. Almost a half of reported cases of HIV infection in the UK are currently in those aged 29 or under. Such global statistics, however, conceal significant local variations. In England, the majority of cases of infection have been reported within three of the four Thames regions amongst young men who have had sex with other men. In Scotland, HIV infection amongst young people is more closely related to injecting drug use, although throughout the UK as a whole transmission through unprotected heterosexual sex is on the increase.

Within country variations such as these are parallelled by differences between countries. In North Western Europe, particularly in Scandinavian countries and in The Netherlands, reported cases of HIV infection amongst young people are most closely linked to sex between men and to injecting drug use, but heterosexual transmission is rising. In Southern European countries such as Italy and Spain reported cases of infection are primarily linked to injecting drug use. The epidemiology of HIV and AIDS in central and eastern European countries such as Hungary and East Germany most closely mirrors that in North Western Europe, whereas that in countries such as Poland is closer to the pattern characteristic in Southern Europe. There are countries of course which have relatively unique epidemiological characteristics — Albania still has no reported cases of infection in any age group, and there are large numbers of reported cases of HIV infection amongst the very young in countries such as the Soviet Union and Romania where transmission has taken place in hospitals and clinics, where infection control procedures have been lax.

Being Young, Being Sexual

Many adults take it for granted that adolescence is a stage of life fraught with difficulties and problems. Adolescents, it seems, are prone to emotional instability, risk taking, sexual experimentation, alcohol abuse and involvement with illicit drugs. Their behaviour is likely to be unpredictable, and their moods and motivations volatile. They cannot be relied upon, nor necessarily do they know their own minds. Such views, widely promoted by medicine and social science since the turn of the century, are uncritically accepted by many involved in health education and health promotion. Rarely is the time taken to pause and consider whether there is any *necessary* correspondence between chronological age, biological maturity and personal and social behaviour.

The origins of these taken-for-granted assumptions can be traced back to late Victorian writing focussing upon the impulsivity and waywardness of youth. They are expressed most eloquently in Stanley Hall's 1905 textbook[6] on adolescence which first characterised the time as a period of storm and stress. Subsequent authors took the view that adolescence is a transcultural, transhistorical and universal phenomenon. As Benedict (1934) put it, it is a state "as definitely characterised by domestic explosions and rebellion, as typhoid is marked by fevers". The work of psychologists such as Freud[7] (1937), and Erikson[8] (1968) were central in consolidating such views. Erikson in particular promoted the view that one of the developmental tasks associated with adolescence is the attainment of a coherent sense of self-identity. Young people, he feared, find it hard to retain a sense of time, encounter difficulties when they need to harness their energies towards the attainment of particular goals, and are prone to rebel when confronted by adults in authority. Whilst modern "lifespan" theories of adolescence begin to acknowledge the diversity of young people's experience, they have done little to ameliorate the impact of these more traditional modes of thought. Thus it is not untypical to read that amongst adolescents "the combination of experimental behaviour and a sense of invincibility contributes to many risks ... peer pressure, role expectations and group norms promote not only sexual experimentation, but also ... behaviour such as sex and alcohol or drug use ... that elevate(s) risk"[9].

In the burgeoning literature on young people and HIV/AIDS, adolescents are most frequently constructed as "unknowledgeable", "overpressured", "developmentally immature", "tragic" or "at high risk". Elsewhere, the implications of this strategy are spelled out in fuller detail[10]. Suffice it to say here they succeed in homogenising and pathologising young people's experience. They suggest that *all* young people are potentially irresponsible and immature, and they marginalise the impact of class, gender, sexuality, disability and cultural differences as they impact upon young people's lives. Such social constructions are therefore less than useful when it comes to planning HIV/AIDS health promotion activities in particular settings and involving specific groups of young people.

A parallel set of problems arises in relation to studies of young people's sexual and reproductive health behaviour. Much of the work in this field begins with negative rather than positive definitions of sexual and reproductive health. Thus, unintended teenage pregnancy and the incidence of STDs amongst young people become the subject of enquiry, rather than sexual pleasure or sexual enjoyment. There is of course relatively little research into the sexual and reproductive health needs of young lesbians and young gay men.

Between 40% and 50% of young people in countries such as France, The Netherlands, Great Britain and the United States have the experience of penetrative (hetero)sexual intercourse by the age of 18[2]. In Britain, a recent national survey showed that seven out of ten 16 year old young men in Britain used a condom when last having penetrative sex. Condom use, however, declines with age, and only five out of ten 19 year olds in the same survey reported using a condom at last intercourse[11].

Condom use is also less likely amongst those who have had four or more sexual partners in the last 12 months[11,12]. In heterosexual relationships, it is the desire to avoid pregnancy rather than STDs which is the major factor influencing the kind of protection young people use. As a result the contraceptive pill is the form of protection most often used by young people of all ages in Britain today. When condoms are used in relationships where the woman is also taking an oral contraceptive, they tend to be used inconsistently. In Weisman *et al's* study[13], only 16% of the young women interviewed, all of whom were taking the contraceptive pill, regularly used condoms as well.

Some measure of the extent to which young people may put themselves at risk through sexual activity is given by statistics on teenage pregnancy, particularly those where conception is followed by termination. In the United States, it has been estimated that 3 in 10 sexually active young women become pregnant during their teenage years. In the United States, too, some 80-90% of pregnancies amongst sexually active 15-19 year old women were unintended[14].

Globally, STD rates are highest amongst those aged 20-24, followed by those aged 15-19 and those aged 25-29[4]. While some young people may be unclear about the ways in which STDs can be avoided, knowledge is not the only thing that matters. Unequal power relationships between young women and young men, for example, make it especially difficult for the former in particular to protect themselves against infection. It is not a simple matter for young women to "insist" that their male partners use condoms when having penetrative sex, or practise non-penetrative sexual activity[15].

HIV/AIDS Health Promotion with Young People

In the light of the preceding comments, health educators and health promoters should adopt a critical stance when planning to meet young people's sexual and reproductive health needs, as well as when working to reduce the transmission of HIV and other STDs. They should be properly sceptical of the suggestion that adolescence is a unitary experience. The transition from childhood to adulthood varies considerably within, as well as between, societies. HIV/AIDS health promotion therefore most appropriately begins with a local needs assessment which identifies the experiences and aspirations of particular groups of young people in specific economic and cultural circumstances. Similarly, work which fails to take seriously the extent to which many young people's sexual and reproductive health choices are influenced by the desire to avoid pregnancy rather than STDs, is likely to be ill-founded. Work to provide for the sexual and reproductive health of young lesbians and young gay men is most notable by its absence, but when it is being planned we should be aware that different principles will apply. In the remainder of this chapter, we will identify some priorities for HIV/AIDS education and health promotion with young people which derive from the issues discussed above. Four key areas of work exist: work to identify young people's health promotion needs, work to evaluate the relevance and appropriateness of peer-led education, work to educate and train teachers and youth workers, and work with politicians, policy makers and the media.

Identifying Needs

When it comes to identifying young people's needs in relations to HIV/AIDS and education for sexual and reproductive health, and when it comes to meeting these, several difficulties can arise. These include how best to carry out enquiry into young people's knowledge, attitudes and beliefs, as well as their past and present sexual behaviour. As many researchers have found, structured questionnaires and interviews are perhaps not the best approach to adopt. Difficulties can arise when framing questions which are both meaningful and relevant. What is more, data gathered from large groups of young people resident within a particular area or neighbourhood may be of little use when it comes to planning specific interventions. It is perhaps better to begin with the expressed needs of young people themselves, accessed via focus group activity or small group discussion in schools, youth clubs and youth centres, than with the findings generated by larger scale surveys. It is essential though, in collecting this kind of information, to provide appropriate guarantees of confidentiality/anonymity if valid responses are to be obtained.

Needs assessments should also identify the sources of information which young people trust. In some circumstances (but not in all), these may be parents or relatives, in others they may be teachers, in yet others they may be peers or the media. There are no hard and fast rules to obey in this respect. Current research fails to suggest that any one of these sources of information is more consistently credible than any other. HIV/AIDS health promotion activity should therefore seek to utilise those channels that are most appropriate to particular groups. These can only be identified after talking with young people themselves and listening carefully to what they have to say.

Adults too have needs in relation to the work they may be asked to carry out. It should not be assumed *a priori* that teachers and/or youth workers have been trained in the necessary skills and techniques, still less can we be sure that their knowledge base is sound and that they will adopt a suitably non-discriminatory approach. Appropriate training packages need to be developed which provide such individuals with the opportunity to assess present knowledge levels, present skills and present attitudes and beliefs. Only then can steps be taken to remedy deficiencies and to re-evaluate unhelpful and prejudicial attitudes and sentiments. It should never be assumed that *all* teachers, youth workers and other adults are well suited to work in this field, and it may be better in some circumstances to accept that HIV/AIDS education and other work to promote sexual and reproductive health is best undertaken only by a few. Such individuals will, however, need support in their relationships with parents, colleagues and friends as well as with young people themselves. Effective work in this field engages strongly with the emotions as issues of life, death, pain, suffering, pleasure, passion, love and desire are brought to the fore.

Evaluating Peer-led Education

There is much talk nowadays of the usefulness of peer-led education in meeting young people's needs. Unfortunately, the term itself describes a multitude of possible interventions. For some, peer-led education must of its essence be a group process, for others it can involve one-to-one work. For some, peer-led education must be involving and participatory, for others it can involve showing videos and giving talks. For some, peer-led education means working from the agendas of scientists, doctors and other "experts", for others it should begin with the needs of young people themselves. Whilst numerous peer-led education projects are under way, few have been evaluated, and whilst this kind of approach may prove useful in some settings, it does not provide all the answers. Health promotion experience suggests that only those strategies which begin with young people's express needs, which are well structured and well supervised, which seek to clarify rather than prescribe, and which involve the use of credible sources of information, are likely to succeed. Whilst this kind of work may prove successful in meeting the needs of "harder to reach" groups such as young gay men, homeless young people etc, its value in other settings may be more limited.

The Training of Teachers, Youth Workers and Other Adults

It is often assumed somewhat unproblematically that teachers and youth workers are well placed to mediate between sources of public information and young people themselves. Whilst some young people may value and respect those adults they meet in school and in youth clubs and in youth centres, it should never be assumed that the adults themselves feel well-equipped to educate about HIV and AIDS. These are not topics which are central within the curriculum offered by teacher and youth work training. Effective education about HIV and AIDS requires clear, coherent and complementary policies in schools and elsewhere about how education for sexual and reproductive health should take place. In many European countries, such policies are currently not in place, and where they are, teachers and youth workers often feel ill equipped to implement them. Work to challenge discrimination and hostility towards gay men, for example, needs to be undertaken with sensitivity and care. It often requires skills and sensitivities which need to be learned beforehand. Similar issues arise in relation to work exploring the nature and consequences of drug use, particularly where substances are injected.

In-service support is also needed by teachers and youth and community educators. This can be provided locally through short courses as well as through the establishment of training support networks. Training forums of this kind can provide opportunities for reflection and evaluation after work with young people has taken place. They can also help in the dissemination of new knowledge and new information. In-service education and training also needs to provide guidance on ways in which popular prejudices can successfully be challenged. Work of this kind often constitutes the "forgotten agenda" in the HIV/AIDS field. It is all too easy to become preoccupied with the "facts" and with allowing young people to explore their attitudes and feelings, whilst forgetting the rights of and our responsibilities towards those already infected and the groups which have been the first to bear the burden of the present epidemic.

Regardless of who undertakes it, HIV/AIDS education should be provided in an integrated and multi-disciplinary way. It is not appropriate in schools, for example, to suggest that this kind of work is the prerogative of the science teacher, or the physical education specialist for that matter. HIV/AIDS articulates with many aspects of life, from those which are narrowly biological to those that concern emotions, feelings and relationships. There are opportunities throughout the curriculum for work on these important matters and this kind of integrated approach is the one most likely to ensure that young people's needs are most adequately met.

Working with Politicians, Policy Makers and the Media

Much of the work pointed to above is likely to fail unless it takes place within an appropriate political and ideological climate. Politicians and policy makers need to be convinced that education for sexual and reproductive health is an important issue. They need to be persuaded moreover that HIV and AIDS cannot and should not be tackled in isolation as topics to be taught on a one-off basis. But putting sexual and reproductive health on the agenda is no easy task. There are those, for example, who believe that to discuss sex is to promote it. There are others who would seek to link any discussion and debate to specific moral agendas. And there are those, it must be admitted, who would prefer it if sex did not exist. But to be influenced by such views is to do young people a grave disservice. It is, moreover, to disempower them in the face of risk. Whilst the aims of politicians, clergy, parents, teachers and youth workers may not always coincide, this should never be used as the basis on which to deny young people the means to minimise the risk. Increasingly, European countries are turning to a pragmatic approach, one which recognises the diversity of ways in which people express themselves sexually, reproductively and emotionally. This kind of strategy is the one most likely to succeed in bringing about and sustaining behaviour change where necessary, and in promoting the maintenance of safer behaviours where such already exist. Work is needed, though, to convince some politicians, some media commentators and all moral entrepreneurs of the necessity of such work, and health educators and health promoters frequently neglect the role they have to play here. Perhaps training in public relations and media liaison should be made more central as a professional development activity. Certainly it is possible to win hearts and minds through HIV/AIDS work so as to create a more appropriate context for activities involving young people.

Acknowledgements

We gratefully acknowledge the assistance and support provided by Mukesh Kapila, Hannah Cinamon, Andrea Young and colleagues at the Health Education Authority in preparing this paper, as well as the contributions of workshop members themselves. Thanks must also go to Malcolm McEachran, Barbara Kenmir and Rita Ward, librarians at Bristol Polytechnic, the Family Planning Association and the International Planned Parenthood Federation respectively.

References

1. Bury J. Teenage pregnancy: the problem hasn't gone away. New York: Guttmacher Institute, 1984.

2. Jones E, Darroch Forrest J, Goldman N, Henshaw S, Lincoln R, Rosoff J, Westoff C, Wulf D. Teenage pregnancy in industrialised countries: a study sponsored by the Allen Guttmacher Institute. New Haven: Yale University Press, 1986.

3. Jones E, Darroch Forrest J, Goldman N, Henshaw S, Lincoln R, Rosoff J, Westoff C, Wulf D. Teenage pregnancy in developed countries: determinants and policy implications. Family Planning Perspectives 1988; **17(2)**: 53-63.

4. World Health Organisation. The health of youth: young people and adults face the issues together. A summary of national and regional activities in preparation for the Technical Discussions and beyond. Facts for action: youth and sexually transmitted diseases. Geneva: WHO, 1989.

5. World Health Organisation. The reproductive health of adolescents: a joint WHO/UNFPA/UNICEF statement. Geneva: World Health Organisation, 1989.

6. Hall S. Adolescence: its psychology and its relations to physiology, anthropology, sociology, sex, crime, religion and education. New York: Appleton, 1905.

7. Freud S. The ego and the mechanisms of defence. London: Hogarth, 1937.

8. Erikson E. Identity, youth and crisis. New York: Norton, 1968.

9. Keeling R. AIDS prevention challenges for colleges and universities. Focus - a guide to AIDS research and counselling 1990; **5(4)**: 1-2.

10. Warwick I, Aggleton P J. Adolescents, young people and AIDS research. *In:* Aggleton P, Davies P, Hart G (Eds). AIDS: individual, cultural and policy dimensions. London: Falmer Press, 1990.

11. MORI. Young adults' health and lifestyles: sexual health. Unpublished study conducted for the Health Education Authority, London, 1990.

12. Ford N, Bowie C. Urban-rural variations in the level of heterosexual activity of young people. AREA 1989; **21(3)**: 237-48.

13. Weisman C S, Plichta S, Nathanson C A, Ensminger M, Robinson J C. Consistency of condom use for disease prevention among adolescent users of oral contraceptives. Family Planning Perspectives 1991; **23(2)**: 71-73.

14. Hayes C D (ed). Risking the future: adolescent sexuality, pregnancy and childbearing, Vol. 1. Washington: National Academy Press, 1987.

15. Holland J, Ramazanoglu C, Scott S, Sharpe S, Thompson, R. Between embarrassment and trust - young women and the diversity of condom use. *In:* Aggleton P, Davies P, Hart G (eds). AIDS: Responses, Interventions and Care. London: Falmer Press, 1991.

13

Promoting Sexual Health: Strategies for Reaching and Empowering Women

Background paper and report by Virginia Blakey, Healthy Sexuality Programme, Health Promotion Authority for Wales, Cardiff.

Other members of the group were:

Sevgi Aral (Chairperson)	*USA*
Susan Biersteker	*The Netherlands*
Lynne Clarke	*UK*
Pilar Estebanez	*Spain*
Sonja Fossum	*Norway*
Christine Höpfner	*Germany*
Torben Jensen	*Denmark*
Hilary Kinnell	*UK*
Susanne Kroon	*Denmark*
Rudolf Mak	*Belgium*
Ruth Morgan Thomas	*UK*
Miriam Nhariwa	*Zimbabwe*
Brigitte Obrist	*Switzerland*
Jorge Santos Cardoso	*Portugal*
Nicola Woodward	*UK*
Yuris Zaltsmanis	*Latvia*

Introduction

Information about the incidence of sexually transmitted diseases (STDs) in Europe is incomplete because of national differences in reporting and collation of statistics. Nevertheless, data compiled by WHO indicate that sexually transmitted infections pose a serious threat to the well-being of women in Europe.

In recent years, health professionals have become increasingly concerned about complications and late sequelae resulting from untreated or inadequately treated STDs: these can include adverse pregnancy outcomes, neonatal and infant infections, pelvic inflammatory disease, ectopic pregnancy, and infertility. Unfortunately, awareness of the implications of these infections is less widespread among women and in the community.

The "classic" STDs for which statistics are collected are syphilis and gonorrhoea. Untreated *gonorrhoea* is still a major cause of infertility among women, particularly in developing countries. For centuries, prior to the discovery of effective treatments in the early 1900s, *syphilis* was regarded with fear because the untreated infection could lead to paralysis, blindness, insanity and ultimately death.

In an overview of STD incidence in Europe, Meheus[1] notes that there was a sharp decline in rates of syphilis and gonorrhoea between World War II and the late 1950s; this was followed by an increase during the 1960s-early 1970s, and then by a further decline from the late 1970s to the present. However, other STDs appear to be increasing. *Chlamydia trachomatis*, for which wide-scale testing techniques became available in the 1970s, is now known to be widespread; chlamydial infections are recognised as a major cause of pelvic inflammatory disease and infertility in women. Incidence and prevalence of *genital herpes*, a painful and often recurrent lifelong condition, have risen dramatically during the last 20 years (in the UK, for example, there was a five-fold increase in incidence between 1970 to 1986, and this was greater among women than among men). The last two decades have also seen an almost exponential increase in the reported incidence of *genital warts*; these are caused by human papilloma virus, which has been associated with cancer of the cervix. The death rate from this cancer among women under 30 in the UK has quadrupled since the late 1960s, and it has been suggested that this is somehow linked to rapid spread of human papilloma virus and genital herpes infection[1].

The most recently identified STD, HIV infection, has been widely publicized, but awareness of its significance for women has been slow to develop in Europe because the infection was initially found almost exclusively among gay men. Women currently represent approximately 12 per cent of the total reported AIDS cases in Europe[2], and incidence is rising; in the UK, for example, AIDS cases among women increased by 78 per cent during 1990. In some major cities in Western Europe, as in parts of the USA and sub-saharan Africa, AIDS is already the leading cause of death for women aged 20-40 years[3]. The possibility of transmission of the infection from mother to baby during pregnancy or birth means that the increasing infection rate among women also has significance for numbers of HIV-infected infants and cases of paediatric AIDS.

Evidence shows that the presence of other STDs increases the risks of sexual transmission of HIV infection. Sexually transmitted diseases that cause genital ulcer disease (including syphilis, genital herpes and chlamydia) have been associated with an increased risk of acquiring HIV infection. Conversely, HIV infection appears to have an adverse effect on symptoms and treatment of other STDs, and thus probably promotes their spread. If, as this implies, HIV and other STDs interact to promote one another's transmission, this vicious circle can best be interrupted by more aggressive control of STDs other than HIV[4].

It is clear that many of the educational messages aimed at reducing the risk of HIV transmission (provision of clear and specific information about risky sexual practices, encouragement of condom use and non-penetrative sexual techniques, development of skills in communicating about sex and negotiating safer sex) are also relevant for general STD prevention, and indeed for other health-related issues of relevance to women such as prevention of unwanted pregnancy. For these reasons, comprehensive prevention strategies which place HIV and other STDs in a broad social context of sexual health may well be more acceptable to women and more successful in achieving their goal. Central to this comprehensive approach should be the concept that sexuality is a potentially pleasurable area of activity which women have the right to enjoy.

Health Promotion Issues for Women

Health promotion for women on issues relating to STDs, particularly HIV, needs to focus on the following issues[5]:

- *Informing women about the risk of sexually transmitted infections, including HIV.* This information needs to be given in a way which enables women to understand how such infections might affect their own lives, and which motivates them to take positive action to protect themselves. It should not be unduly alarmist, but should help women to make a realistic assessment of ways in which they may be at risk.

- *Helping women to take more control in a heterosexual partnership than is traditionally expected.* Women need to be able to negotiate safer sex where there is a possible risk of HIV infection; this may mean using condoms, or choosing the option of no sex or non-penetrative sex.

- *Informing sexually active women of child-bearing age about:*

   Transmission risks to their child during pregnancy, birth and through breast milk;

   The *effect of pregnancy* on HIV infection;

   The advantages and disadvantages of *anonymised and voluntary ante-natal HIV antibody testing.*

- *Informing women in a supportive way about the risk of HIV transmission through injecting drug use,* and offering help in adopting safer injecting practices or coming off drugs.

- *Providing women with information about available services, sources of advice and support, and self-help measures such as changes in life-style which can reduce risk and promote health.*

However, it must be recognised that the behaviour changes which information campaigns aim to promote pose some formidable challenges. There are many deeply-rooted social and cultural constraints which hinder the implementation of prevention campaigns and which make it very difficult for individual women to adopt safer behaviours: indeed, as Cochran[6] states, "Preventive behaviours can be a luxury to be afforded only if they do not conflict with other primary needs". The following examples highlight some specific difficulties affecting particular groups of women:

Young women

Societies are often reluctant to recognise that young women are sexually active: parents and schools may prefer to moralise rather than give factual information and practical help. There may be legislation which limits the form and content of education on sexuality-related issues.

Even where young women have access to information about safer sex, they may still find it difficult to put their knowledge into practice. Romantic ideas may override awareness of the risks; "serious relationships" may be seen as a defence against HIV and other sexually transmitted diseases, and "love is not having to use a condom". Male attitudes may also undermine attempts to practise safer sex: a young woman who carries condoms and advocates their use is still liable to be labelled as a "slag" or an "easy lay". Health promotion programmes need to recognise that young women's sexual relationships take place within a social context shaped by male dominance, where they may be relatively powerless to insist on safer sex[7,8,9].

Cultural taboos and social vulnerability

It is not only young women who are affected by wider social and cultural constraints. Women from particular ethnic, religious and cultural groups may be influenced by social norms which make it difficult to communicate with male partners about sexual practices or to take independent action on these issues. Problems of language, literacy, access, and the attitudes of health professionals may make it difficult for women to make contact with preventive and treatment services.

Women sex workers

Since the onset of HIV, sex workers have been linked with gay men and drug users as the focus of moral panic about the epidemic. In fact, available evidence from Europe suggests that women sex workers in general are not currently experiencing high levels of HIV infection, although they may experience high levels of other STDs. Many sex workers were already using condoms to prevent STD transmission before the advent of HIV infection; with increasing awareness about HIV and AIDS, condom use has increased still further, and sex workers are now acting as HIV educators to their clients. In those European cities such as Barcelona, Frankfurt and Milan where HIV rates are significant among sex workers, the main risk factor is sharing of injecting equipment[10,11].

In terms of sexual transmission, sex workers themselves are at risk from clients who refuse to use condoms. Many women sex workers may also prefer not to use condoms with lovers or husbands, as a way of distinguishing between work and their private life. In this respect, they face similar problems to other women in terms of negotiating safer sex in a long-term relationship. However, ignorance and prejudice about the realities of sex work on the part of officials and the general public means that prevention campaigns often do not take account of these factors. These judgemental attitudes may also deter sex workers from approaching services which have a role in promoting sexual health.

Legislation relating to prostitution can also place barriers in the way of HIV prevention work. Experts from a number of European countries have argued that decriminalisation of prostitution may be necessary in situations where laws are ineffective or counterproductive[12].

Injecting drug use and women

Evaluation of harm minimization approaches suggest that drug users are adopting safer injecting practices in response to the threat of HIV infection. However, the same research also shows that *women drug users* are under-represented among needle exchange clients[13]. In addition, it is clear that injecting drug users find it much easier to change their injecting practices than their sexual practices[14,15,16]. Many women drug users are emotionally and economically dependent, socially isolated and lacking in self-esteem. Practising safer sex may pose a substantial challenge, as it may be difficult or indeed dangerous for women in this situation to attempt to persuade their partners of the need to change their sexual behaviour. This poses significant problems for STD prevention efforts[17]. Similar considerations may apply to *female partners of injecting drug users*. British studies suggest that many male injecting drug users choose sexual partners who do not inject, in order to reduce their own risk of HIV transmission[14,18,19]. In spite of adoption of safer sex and safer drug use practices by many male drug users, there may be an increased possibility of HIV transmission from male drug injectors to women who do not inject drugs in areas of higher seropositivity among drug users.

Women who have sex with women

Initial lesbian concerns around HIV infection focussed on the social and political impact of the virus on the gay and lesbian community; the main health promotion task was to overcome public prejudice and misconceptions about HIV, including the labelling of lesbians as a "risk group". Many lesbians assumed that sex between women was safer sex, and health care workers shared this view. However, as knowledge about the virus has increased, it has become clear that some lesbian sexual practices can carry a risk of transmission of HIV and other STDs. Lesbian women need appropriate information on safer sex practices[20,21]. Provision of education in this area, particularly to young women, may be hampered by public attitudes and legislation which inhibit discussion of sexual orientation.

Female partners of bisexual men

Women whose partners have sex with both women and men may be particularly at risk of HIV infection and other STDs. A preliminary British study[22] suggests that, while many bisexual men have adopted safer sex practices with their male partners, the great majority of those with female partners are continuing to have unprotected intercourse with them and so potentially put them at risk of infection. Women in this situation are hard to identify, either because they are not aware of their partner's activities or because they are reluctant to acknowledge them. Designing and implementing appropriate prevention programmes is therefore a particularly challenging task, involving greater openness about the varied nature of sexuality and sexual behaviour.

Reproductive rights

Partner notification relating to STDs is of vital concern to women, because of possible infertility resulting from infections and the implications of this for future childbearing intentions. Because of the complex medical, social, legal and ethical issues raised by partner notification (particularly in relation to HIV infection), guidelines in this area need to be especially sensitive and to respect the rights and dignity of both the index patient and their partners[23].

HIV antibody testing as a public health measure is of particular significance to women because of the growing trend towards routine *mass screening programmes for pregnant women*. The appropriate uses of such testing are widely debated. Many health professionals consider that, with evolving experience of the use of preventive drugs, there are medical advantages in an early awareness of positivity status (although the low representation of women, particularly pregnant women, in clinical trials means that data relating to women are limited). Others argue that the stigma and social disadvantages which can result from a positive test result (eg. the possibility that the child of a drug-using mother might be taken into care) may deter women from attending pre-natal services where testing is likely to take place. It is most important that testing should take place only on a voluntary basis with informed consent, and also with supportive pre- and post-test counselling and assurances of confidentiality. Where mass screening takes place, questions may legitimately be raised about the quality of counselling.

HIV testing of pregnant women is also significant because it is linked to the issue of perinatal transmission, and this in turn is linked to *abortion counselling*. Women who receive positive HIV test results may find that some health professionals question their right to continue with the pregnancy, although studies have shown that many women with HIV infection do not see this as a reason for termination[24]. For some women, the positive values attached to motherhood may outweigh other considerations. Evolving knowledge about the relative risk of perinatal transmission of HIV infection has shown that earlier assessments of the probability of transmission were possibly too high[25], and that factors such as the timing of pregnancy in relation to the stage of the infection may be significant. As knowledge of these issues develops, it is important that it is made available to women so that they can make informed decisions. Policy-makers need to ensure that counselling in this area does not infringe the personal reproductive rights of the women concerned[2]. In addition, improved access to abortion services within the statutory health sector is vital to ensure that women who choose this option do not experience unnecessary delays.

Health Promotion Experience

As with other areas of health promotion, many projects focussing on women and sexual health are not formally evaluated, and more effort needs to go into dissemination of findings. The following are some examples of projects and approaches which may be appropriate for promoting sexual health among women.

Young people are often very receptive to *information campaigns* on a topic which is of concern to them. In 1986 the *Swedish Association for Sex Education (RFSU)* designed a booklet entitled "How to live your life without being hassled by AIDS, herpes, condyloma, chlamydia or gonorrhoea" which was personally addressed and sent out to all young people in Stockholm aged 18-24. A follow-up evaluation found that the magazine was highly rated for information, relevance, and credibility, and 46 per cent of the sample interviewed had kept it for reference[26].

Many commercial and voluntary organizations use *T-shirt slogans* to raise awareness and get publicity for their product or cause, and this approach can also be adopted to promote sexual health. *The Family Planning Association of New South Wales*, Australia has produced a T-shirt featuring the slogan "Condoms are a girl's best friend", which is selling well among young women.

Mass media advertising to encourage condom use helps to create a supportive public environment for changes to safer sex practices by individual women and their partners. National health promotion agencies and AIDS agencies in a number of countries (including Germany, Spain and the UK) have run television and cinema campaigns along these lines. "Safer sex" has also featured as a theme in *soap operas* in several countries.

Empowerment is a key issue in *community-based education projects* for women. In England, the *Health Education Authority* is currently funding a study to look at resources and training in assertiveness in the context of women's health education[27]. These lessons are being applied at a grassroots level; the *Girls' and Young Women's Health Project* in North Manchester, England, has involved a group of young women in planning a well women's clinic to meet their specific needs[28].

Experience from Los Angeles suggests[29] that *peer education approaches* can be an effective way of carrying out education work on sexuality-related issues. In this project, young people from a range of cultural backgrounds were trained to do outreach education work with street kids. In a similar project in Brooklyn, New York, the peer educators were also trained in improvisational theatre techniques to increase the impact of their work[30]. While these projects worked with young people of both sexes, the approach could also be used in work specifically with young women.

Where *prostitutes' rights campaigns* exist, these can often provide an excellent base for STD prevention activities among sex workers and their clients. For example, the *Red Thread Organization* in Amsterdam, *CALPEP (the California Prostitutes Education Project)* and the *Prostitutes Collective of Victoria*, Australia, all use their own street outreach workers to distribute condoms and carry out education on safer sex and safer drug use[31,32,33]. Red Thread have also produced a sticker, "Ik doe het met..." — "I do it with (a condom)", which is being prmoted as a slogan not only by sex workers but by anyone who has more than one partner.

Many sex workers are reluctant to approach health services because of fears about encountering judgemental attitudes from health professionals. There is a need to set up *low-threshold services* which can provide basic health care, including STD checks and advice on contraception, as well as information and supplies for safer sex and safer drug use. In Utrecht, The Netherlands, a caravan providing a range of facilities has been situated in the area where many sex workers are based; this has been successful in attracting sex workers and providing a focus for STD prevention activities. Drop-in centres for sex workers along similar lines have been set up in Glasgow, Birmingham, Madrid and other European cities.

Women drug users are often particularly vulnerable and lacking in self-esteem. Education on STD prevention for this group needs to be empowering and to take place within a context of genuine concern for the well-being of the woman. Projects that look at women's broader health needs as well as STD prevention, and which involve the women themselves in the development and delivery of their own education programmes, may be more likely to succeed. A good example of such a project is the *ADAPT programme* in New York, which has had considerable success with street-level education involving distribution of bleach and condoms and helping users to gain access to medical and drug treatment services.

More needs to be done to meet the specific needs of HIV-positive women. The UK organisation *Positively Women,* started by a small group of women with HIV, is addressing these emotional and practical needs through a self-help approach which has included the setting-up of support groups, development of information materials, and advocacy work on behalf of HIV-positive women[34].

While much can be gained from innovative projects and approaches, they are not a replacement for *basic education and health services.* It is vital that resources and staffing of schools, clinics and health centres are maintained so that the preventive and health promotion work carried out in these settings is of a high standard. A *multi-agency approach* to STD education and prevention will ensure that the different sectors are working to a shared agenda and that health promotion efforts make the maximum impact.

Recommendations for Action

On the basis of the issues discussed above, the Working Group made the following recommendations, drawing on the framework of the Ottawa Charter:

Building healthy public policy:

- Greater *involvement of women at policy-making levels,* so that policies and services are more sensitive to the particular needs of women.

- The removal of *legislative barriers* which hinder the provision of factual, non-judgmental *education on sexuality and sexual health* to young women in schools and other youth settings.

- In accordance with the belief that HIV/AIDS is a greater threat to individual and public health than drug misuse, the repeal of *legislation relating to the control of drugs* which hinders effective health promotion and HIV prevention for drug users and their partners.

- The repeal of *legislation relating to prostitution* which hinders the promotion of safer sex education and practice among sex workers.

- Better *integration of the range of services concerned with promoting sexual health,* to achieve a more coordinated and user-friendly approach.

Creating a supportive environment:

- Development of *public education campaigns* to raise public awareness, increase understanding and promote safer sexual behaviours. These should use techniques and formats which are culturally appropriate and suited to the content and complexity of the messages being transmitted; they should not emphasise mass media to the exclusion of other more community-based educational approaches. The aims of the campaign should be:

    1) to break down the public misapprehensions and prejudice surrounding sexually transmitted diseases and perceived "risk groups" (eg sex workers, foreign women);

    2) to create a more sympathetic and caring attitude towards all people with STDs, particularly those with HIV/AIDS;

    3) to continue to highlight the risks of HIV infection for women, and to start to highlight other STDs;

    4) to emphasise the need for safer sex behaviours among men who have sex with women;

    5) to present a more erotic image of safer sex, including condom use.

- Greater *social marketing of condoms* to ensure easy availability and access for all, including women.

Strengthening community action:

- Provision of *financial support from the statutory sector to womens' groups* to enable them to develop their own educational and advocacy work on issues related to prevention of sexually transmitted diseases and promotion of sexual health. Groups which have a role to play would include formal and informal groups with an interest in women's health, including self-help groups focussing on specific issues (eg. herpes, infertility); groups representing HIV seropositive women; prostitutes' collectives; organisations concerned with the particular needs of women from different cultural and religious minorities; and organisations for women with other special needs (eg. hearing-impaired women). Groups whose formal and informal networks are not well developed (eg. women drug users and women partners of drug users) may need particular support.

Developing personal skills:

- Support for the *economic and legal empowerment of women,* which the Working Group saw as fundamental to efforts to improve women's skills and self-esteem.

- Development of appropriate *educational programmes on sexuality and sexual health* in schools and other community settings. The *content* of these programmes should be factual, non-judgemental, and presented in a form which is accessible and culturally appropriate (though cultural disapproval of sex education should not be used to deny women access to such programmes). Education should cover values, attitudes, self-esteem and self-empowerment as well as factual information and familiarisation with appropriate services. It should emphasise the pleasurable potential of sex as well as the need to avoid risky practices. The *format* should be participatory rather than didactic; it should include the opportunity to practise appropriate skills such as negotiating safer sex. For some groups, programmes may be most effective when based on an outreach or peer-led approach.

- Even with education and empowerment, many women will still be constrained by the attitudes of their male partners, who will often hold the balance of power in a relationship. It is vital that educational programmes are targetted at *men who have sex with women.* Future workshops of this kind should include a specific working group to consider the particular barriers and constraints operating in this area.

Reorienting services:

- *Raise the profile and status of services related to sexually transmitted diseases.* In most European countries, the increase in demand for testing, diagnosis and counselling for HIV infection has highlighted a general need to invest more resources in these services.

- *Improve accessibility and "user-friendliness" of services relating to sexual health.* Education is needed to make all those health professionals who are dealing with women in the context of sexual health — general practitioners, family planning clinic staff, STD specialists — less judgemental and more sensitive to the needs of the women who approach them. Particular emphasis should be placed on the skills needed for working with young women.

- Provide *better training for health professionals* working in this area, both in terms of the general degree of comfort and confidence which they feel when discussing sexuality-related issues, and in improving specific skills such as taking sexual histories and risk-assessment/risk-reduction counselling.

- Encourage health professionals to recognise that they have an *advocacy role* in relation to opinion leaders and the general public, and that this should be used to publicise the particular needs of women in the area of sexual health.

- Ensure that *HIV testing of women* is carried out on a voluntary, confidential basis with confirmed consent, and that the counselling given is sensitive to women's needs and does not infringe the personal reproductive rights of the women involved.

- *Promote research by women for women on aspects of HIV and other sexually transmitted diseases.* Areas requiring more detailed research include surveillance data for STDs in general; more detailed information on the implications of STDs for women; and specific studies on transmission, diagnosis, treatment and progression of HIV in women, including issues relating to pregnancy.

References

1. Meheus A. The spectrum of sexually transmitted diseases and approaches for their control. *In:* Paalman M (ed). Promoting safer sex. Amsterdam: Swets and Zeitlinger, 1990, 17-24.

2. Hankins C A. Issues involving women, children and AIDS primarily in the developed world. J Acquired Immune Deficiency Syndromes 1990; **3(4)**: 443-48.

3. Chin J. Current and future dimensions of the HIV/AIDS pandemic in women and children. Lancet 1990; **336**: 221-24.

4. Aral S O, Holmes K K. Sexually transmitted diseases in the AIDS era. Scientific American 1991; **264(2)**: 18-25.

5. Wellings K. Women and AIDS. AIDS Programme Papers 5. London: Health Education Authority, 1989.

6. Cochran S D. Women and HIV infection: issues in prevention and behaviour change. *In:* Mays V M, Albee G W, Schneider S F (eds). Primary prevention of AIDS. Newbury Park: Sage, 1989.

7. Holland J, Ramazanoglu C, Scott S, Sharpe S, Thomson R. Sex, gender and power: young women's sexuality in the shadow of AIDS. Sociology of Health & Illness 1990; **12(3)**: 336-50.

8. Holly L. "It makes you think again": discussing AIDS and other sexually transmitted diseases. *In:* Holly L (ed). Girls and Sexuality. Milton Keynes: Open University Press, 1989, 25-37.

9. Richardson D. AIDS education and women: sexual and reproductive issues. *In:* Aggleton P, Davies P, Hart G (eds). AIDS: individual, cultural and policy dimensions. London: Falmer Press, 1990.

10. Padian N S. Prostitute women and AIDS: epidemiology. AIDS 1988; **2(6)**: 413-19.

11. Plant M. AIDS, drugs and prostitution. London: Tavistock/Routledge, 1990.

12. Biersteker S. Promoting safer sex in prostitution: impediments and opportunities. *In:* Paalman M. (ed). Promoting safer sex. Amsterdam: Swets and Zeitlinger, 1990, 143-52.

13. Stimson G V, Donoghoe M C, Lart R, Dolan K. Distributing sterile needles and syringes to people who inject drugs: the syringe-exchange experiment. *In:* Strang J, Stimson G V (eds). AIDS and drug misuse. London: Routledge, 1990, 222-31.

14. Donoghoe M C, Stimson G V, Dolan K A. Sexual behaviour of injecting drug users and associated risks of HIV infection for non-injecting sexual partners. AIDS Care 1989; **1(1)**: 51-58.

15. Kall K I, Olin R G. HIV status and changes in risk behaviour among intravenous drug users in Stockholm 1987-88. AIDS 1990; **4(2)**: 153-157.

16. Van den Hoek A, Van Haastrecht H, Coutinho R. Heterosexual behaviour of intravenous drug users in Amsterdam: implications for the AIDS epidemic. AIDS 1990; **4(5)**: 449-453.

17. Worth D. Sexual decision-making and AIDS: why condom promotion among vulnerable women is likely to fail. Studies in Family Planning 1989; **20(6)**: 297-307.

18. Klee H, Faugier J, Hayes C, Boulton T, Morris J. Sexual partners of injecting drug users: the risk of HIV infection. Br J Addiction 1990; **85(3)**: 413-418.

19. McKeganey N, Barnard M, Watson H. HIV-related risk behaviour among a non-clinic sample of injecting drug users. Br J Addiction 1989; **84(12)**: 1481-90.

20. Adams M L. All that rubber, all that talk: lesbians and safer sex. *In:* Reider I, Ruppelt P (eds). Matters of life and death: women speak about AIDS. London: Virago, 1989.

21. Patton C, Kelly J. Making it: a woman's guide to sex in the age of AIDS. Ithaca, New York: Firebrand Books, 1987.

22. Boulton M, Evans Z S, Fitzpatrick R, Hart G. Bisexual men: women, safer sex and HIV transmission. *In:* Aggleton P, Hart G, Davies P (eds). AIDS: responses, interventions and care. London: Falmer Press, 1991, 65-78.

23. World Health Organization Global Programme on AIDS. Consensus statement from consultation on partner notification for preventing HIV transmission (WHO/GPA/INF/89.3). Geneva: WHO, 1989.

24. Johnstone F D, Brettle R P, MacCallum L R, Mok J, Peutherer J F, Burns S. Women's knowledge of their HIV antibody state: its effects on their decision whether to continue the pregnancy. Br Med J 1990; **300**: 23-24.

25. European Collaborative Study. Children born to women with HIV-1 infection: natural history and risk of transmission. Lancet 1991; **337**: 253-60.

26. Fant M. Strategies for national campaigns. Paper presented at Fourth International Conference on AIDS, Stockholm 1988 (6065).

27. Whitehead C. Assertiveness and women's health education: a study to ascertain current resources and training. London: Health Education Authority, 1990.

28. Long S. Girls' and young women's health project. Women's Health Network News 1990; **March**: 3.

29. Arnold W., Barnes F. Peer education program reaches high risk adolescents with AIDS information and prevention. Paper presented at Fifth International Conference on AIDS, Montreal, 1989 (TDO26).

30. Troutman A, Hall J Y. Sex, drugs and AIDS: two innovative approaches to HIV/AIDS prevention education and outreach for minority adolescents. Paper presented at Fifth International Conference, on AIDS, Montreal 1989 (MDO11).

31. AIDSCOM. The Red Thread: the Netherlands. *In:* Education and evaluation: partners in AIDS prevention. Washington: Academy for Educational Development, 1989.

32. Alexander P. Prostitutes prevent AIDS: a manual for health education. San Francisco: California Prostitutes Education Project, 1988.

33. Overs C, Hunter A. AIDS prevention in the legalized sex industry. Paper presented at Fifth International Conference on AIDS, Montreal, 1989 (ThDP91).

34. Thomson K. Self-help: the example of Positively Women. *In:* Henderson S (ed). Women, HIV and drugs: practical issues. London: Institute for the Study of Drug Dependence, 1990, 17-22.

14

Men who have Sex with Men

Background paper and report by Peter Davies, Department of Sociology, University of Essex

Other working group members were:

George Svéd (Chairperson)	Sweden
Sue Bandcroft	UK
Rumen Bostandjiev	Bulgaria
Maurice Cramers	Belgium
Gary Dowsett	Australia
Hans Elbers	The Netherlands
Gunther Grau	Germany
Jakob Haff	Denmark
Robert Hubers	The Netherlands
Edward King	UK
Michael McGovern	UK
Øyvin Palm	Norway
Richard Průša	Czechoslovakia
Michael Quinlan	Republic of Ireland
Theo Sandfort	The Netherlands
Martien Sleutjes	The Netherlands
Hans Peter Waltisberg	Switzerland
Simon Watney	UK
David Wiseman	UK

Introduction

In principle, the state has a responsibility for the health of all its citizens. In practice, access to health care is not equal, but differentially available to those in positions of economic, social or normative superiority. The appearance of AIDS and its spread along lines of social disjunction has dramatised and exacerbated these inequalities.

The distinguished historian Jeffrey Weeks has called AIDS "an epidemic waiting to happen". The early pattern of spread of AIDS and of HIV was one which fell, almost miraculously, into the moral agenda of the emergent "New Right". Predominantly effecting those three shibboleths of 1960s liberalism, women, black people and gay men, AIDS was used by many to justify repressive and reactionary moral and political agenda. Even among liberal state agencies there has been widespread unease at promoting, or being seen to promote reactions to HIV other than those which are consonant with traditional, (hetero)sexual monogamy and fidelity.

Apart from The Netherlands, state responses to AIDS did not begin until 1985-6-7. Prior to that date, only those countries which boasted a gay consciousness and social infrastructure produced effective information and prevention initiatives. Those countries where "gay liberation" movements of the 1960s and 1970s had not had an impact were noticeably tardy in putting together a coherent set of responses to AIDS. It is noticeable even today that the two countries in the EC without large gay communities, Greece and Portugal, have yet to develop AIDS-related organisations. The role of the gay communities in defining, articulating and promulgating an effective, responsible and comprehensive set of responses to AIDS in general and to safer sex in particular must be recognised and respected by state-sponsored programmes.

The gay communities themselves were not and are not of one mind about their response to AIDS. The epidemic has forced gay men into an uneasy and ironic rapprochement with the medical establishment: ironic because it was from the objectification of medical theories that gay movements sought to liberate themselves with a claim to an autochthonous, authentic and autonomic experience. The relationship between these two groups has been uneasy in that gay community-based activists have systematically and specifically challenged traditional medical approaches to prophylaxis, treatment and the testing of drugs. More generally, the homophobia of some medics and other influential individuals and of some national and local organisations and institutions remains a problem. Within the gay communities, there has also been disagreement about what might be termed "sex-negative" and "sex-positive" responses.

The history of the AIDS epidemic has shown that the gay communities, gay men and lesbians together, have created new models of health promotion, innovative approaches to primary and secondary prevention — in particular and most notably creating the notion of safe(r) sex and new models of care and support for people living with HIV and AIDS. In particular, at the start of the epidemic, while state agencies were largely silent, the same communities challenged medical orthodoxy, creating new and adapting old organisations, affiliations and networks to put these ideas into effective practice.

Today, at the start of the second decade of AIDS, these efforts are being systematically excluded from official histories of AIDS. Histories typically begin with a description of state responses, while in the memory of many of us who were involved in the early years of AIDS such responses were the "end of the beginning" of AIDS. Throughout northern Europe, certainly, cases of AIDS began to appear in the very early 1980s, typically 1981-2, gay community organisations emerge soon afterwards and state responses do not begin until about 1985/86. It is not only an offence against history that such a distortion should be allowed, but an insult to the memories of those who fought against and, in many cases, died because of state indifference in the early years.

The Second Decade

In the view of the group, two issues are crucial at the start of the second decade of the epidemic as far as homosexual transmission is involved. First, the increasing and encroaching use of the term "men who have sex with men" and secondly, the threat posed by the use of the term and concept "relapse".

Men who have sex with men

There is no doubt that the phrase "men who have sex with men" is an accurate description of the group which is potentially at risk of transmitting HIV through male-male sexual contact. It is, in this sense, an epidemiological category and, rightly, recognises the fact the sexual behaviour and sexual identity are not co-terminous. The use of the term marks an important stage in the development of state reaction to AIDS in distinguishing the epidemiological category from that of community commitment. Its introduction stemmed partly from the gay communities' work in educating others to acknowledge this distinction.

However, its near universal use, sometimes, wrongly, as a synonym for gay, tends to down-play the past and potential contribution of organisations, individuals and groups from the gay communities. While the distinction between the group "men who have sex with men" and "gay men" is fundamental, the difference is crucial in understanding the different patterns of potential spread of HIV and of effective health promotion. Focussing on "men who have sex with men" as an epidemiological category and the gay communities as engines of health promotion is of some use in clarifying the social processes which affect the spread of HIV.

It is not, however, sufficient. The phrase "men who have sex with men", even as an epidemiological category, fails to acknowledge the diversity of social identities, sexual interactions and structural inequalities that characterise sexual expression. Crucially, it fails to recognise the potential of gay community initiatives in promoting the sexual health of this diverse group. As we have noted, the history of the epidemic shows that the gay communities are effective in defining and putting into practice effective reactions to the problems thrown up by AIDS. The communities themselves, simply by their existence, encourage and generate responses. They have been effective in promoting successful behaviour change at the individual level by fostering self-esteem. A confident gay man in control of his sexuality is more likely to seek out, to heed and to act upon safer sexual practices than a man whose homosexuality is problematic and whose homosexual activity is secretive.

Moreover, gay communities have succeeded, by and large, and in the face of necessity, in creating a culture where safer sex is expected, enforced and reinforced. The normative consensus within the gay communities on the need for safer sex stands in stark and welcome contrast to the continuing denial among most of the heterosexually active and the population at large. There is no doubt that a community united simply by a recognition of its sexual desire is uniquely able to discuss, understand and change sexual behaviour.

Thus, the gay communities are not a "target group" for health promotion by agencies of the state, but an infrastructure for the delivery of health promotion services, messages and interventions effectively and efficiently both to gay men and to the wider population of men who have sex with men.

While the original gay liberation movements of the early 1970s were a part of the "counter-culture", their growth since then has created a complex of institutions and sub-groups of great diversity and energy. Throughout Europe, however, gay communities remain marginal and the focus of much hostility. It is important to encourage governments to decriminalise homosexual behaviour between men and to condemn discrimination on the basis of sexual orientation or behaviour as a matter of public health as well as one of human rights. Countries where gay communities are actually or almost non-existent should encourage the creation of gay social venues as a space where gay consciousness and communities can develop.

Relapse

Our second concern at this point of the epidemic is the use of the term "relapse". It is now generally, though sometimes grudgingly, accepted that the response of men who have sex with men to AIDS has resulted in a significant, perhaps unprecedented, change in sexual behaviour and a subsequent limitation of the spread of the virus through male-male sexual contact. Recently, there has been evidence that the incidence of unsafe sexual behaviour, specifically anal intercourse, is increasing. There have also been reports of rises in the rates of STDs among men who have sex with men, along with some evidence of an increase in the rate of spread of HIV. Some American scientists have sought to interpret this as evidence of "relapse". Many Europeans have, been less happy with this interpretation. It is the strong opinion of the group that the term "relapse" and the theoretical apparatus that lies behind it are unhelpful and dangerous.

First, it is unhelpful as a description of what is happening. We believe that the reasons behind the rise in STDs and reported HIV infection are far more complex than a simple model of "relapse" allows. Part of the increase is certainly to be accounted for by changes in testing policy by physicians. Increases in some STDs are consonant with safe behaviour from the point of view of HIV transmission. Secondly, and specifically, it is unhelpful in focussing attention on the behaviour of the individual and in doing this through the addiction model. This is profoundly insulting; sex is simply not a "bad habit" into which we fall because we cannot help ourselves. More than that, "relapse" as a concept pathologises not only the behaviour but the individual. It resurrects the image of the homosexual man as victim of his biology that gay liberation sought, successfully, to eradicate.

The use of the term relapse is dangerous because it sees sexual behaviour as pathological and those individuals who engage in anal intercourse as mad, bad and dangerous to know. As such it fuels anti-gay prejudice and lends justification to those who would pin the blame for the epidemic on gay men. It is dangerous because it encourages the creation of programmes of therapy on addiction models: twelve step programmes. While such programmes may be of use to a few men, addiction models are simply inappropriate for most men at this stage of the epidemic. As gay men evolve more and more sophisticated strategies of combining safe sex with exciting sex, the aridity of explanatory models and preventive programmes which focus on simple but specious single behaviours becomes increasingly apparent.

Emerging Issues that Face Gay Community Programmes Include:

- *The promotion of general and specific health for people living with HIV and HIV disease*

It is distressingly common for health promotion initiatives to concentrate exclusively or predominantly on the needs of those who are HIV seronegative. Programmes which neither write out nor denigrate those living with HIV serve not only to promote their physical well-being but also to remind others of their rights and needs as individuals and as citizens.

- *Relations with and support for male sex workers*

The gay communities, certainly in their public faces, have been ambivalent on the question of male sex-workers. The existence of sex-workers, particularly those who do not identify as gay, has been seen as inimical to the creation of a gay consciousness and to what is seen as the proper concerns of a gay community. It is, however, a matter of urgency that programmes which address the real needs of sex workers can be initiated, encouraged and maintained. In a few cases, this can be done through the gay communities as a form of outreach. In other cases, and more appropriately, the existing infra-structures of sex work should be enabled and empowered to encourage safer sex and other appropriate changes at the individual and the community level.

- *Issues of drug and alcohol use, and their problematic relationship with safer sex*

There is much simplistic analysis of the relationship between alcohol and drug use and sexual behaviour. There is an urgent need for an informed and rational perspective on these matters.

- *Patterns of social and cultural inequality within the gay communities and the wider group of men who have sex with men*

The diversity of the gay communities is at the heart of this discussion, yet the most public face and voice of the communities in most of the West is the middle-class, articulate, white gay man. It should be recognised that these communities include other groups and individuals whose needs may differ from those of the central group. Groups defined by ethnic background, class and education are the most immediate and pressing priority.

In some cases, existing networks of communication and social exchange can, at least in principle, be used to disseminate information and to initiate and validate health-promoting behaviours. Organisations within minority linguistic, cultural or ethnic groups can, in principle, be used though some cultural traditions are even less accepting of male-male sexual contact than Judaeo-Christian, white European culture. In others, male-male contact is relatively common and accepted within traditional contexts although the label and identity "gay" is unknown or unacknowledged.

It is important that programmes of information aimed at the "general population" include reference to these groups and to others which do not cohere into social networks. There is a dual purpose to such a strategy: to inform the non-gay men who have sex with men of the range of options available to them; and to inform the remainder of the population of the existence and authentic experience of men who have sex with men. Doubtless, such strategies will have to avoid presenting HIV as a problem solely for gay men but this can be done.

There is an general trend in Europe and beyond for funds and programmes specifically directed towards the problems of AIDS to be taken into the mainstream of health care and health promotion, from which they have hitherto been separately funded and managed. While some of the basic work now being undertaken by gay communities can be "mainstreamed", such a move is likely to be neither cost-effective nor practically successful for many important activities. For example, who but gay men are going to form the core of those who undertake work with men who have sex with men in semi-public places?

Conclusion

The challenge to gay community programmes and to state agencies charged with the public health is to initiate, develop and maintain co-operative research which identifies the real reasons for the reported rise in STDs, in particular the increasingly complex strategies that couples are evolving to make their sex lives more fulfilling and more safe. They should take up the challenge of promulgating such information in programmes that are sex-positive, accessible and relevant.

The perspective of this group, is perhaps different from the others represented here. Gay men find it hard to regard the state and the medical profession as unequivocally benign. We look to health professionals for health services that recognise, acknowledge and empower our individual experience, collective history and cultural autonomy. We expect, as of right, not on sufferance, to be involved at every level in the conception, production and delivery of health promotion programmes for our communities and we offer, in return, our collective experience in coping with AIDS and HIV over a decade.

There will be those among the readers of this chapter who think that it merely plays games with words; taking issue with the meaning of words as an exercise in scholastic futility. It will be thought by some that the unfortunate connotations of "relapse", for example, can be avoided by using synonyms or near synonyms, such as the strikingly inelegant "reverse behaviour change". We seek, however, to take issue with the stack of meanings which lie behind the words, the set of demeaning and derogatory attitudes that underpin their use and popularity. We remember that perhaps the single most crucial act in the gay liberation movements of the 1970s was the invention of a self-created and validated term for ourselves: the term gay, which replaced the pathological pigeon-hole into which the medical orthodoxy of the late nineteenth century had thrust us. With this in mind, we recognise that words have power to shape and change the world and in this chapter, we describe the world as we see it. Above all, we refuse to regard sex in general and sex between men in particular as something to be discouraged, grudgingly accepted and indulged in late at night, in the dark and in secret. Rather we believe sex should be encouraged, enjoyed and celebrated and that this sense of delight should be emphasised in the time of AIDS, not denied.

15

Drug Users

Background paper and report by Hugh Dufficy, Deputy Director, SCODA (Standing Conference on Drug Abuse), London

Other members of the group were:

Anne-Lise Middelthon (chairperson)	*Norway*
Judith Baines	*UK*
Christopher Carne	*UK*
Saulius Čaplinskas	*Lithuania*
István Erdélyi	*Hungary*
Umberto Galvan	*Italy*
Louise Hanson	*UK*
Herman Knabe	*Sweden*
Ruth Lowbury	*UK*
Raúl Ortiz de Lejarazu	*Spain*
Louise Pomeroy	*Republic of Ireland*
Daniel Zulaica	*Spain*

Introduction

This report is specifically concerned with the needs of people who use illicit drugs. The participants in this working group came from a wide range of countries throughout Europe including delegates from the Eastern and Central European countries. All participants either worked directly with drug users or were involved in the development of policy issues relating to drug use, in their country or organisation.

Drug Users

Drug users come from all walks of life, cutting across class, race, gender and sexual orientation categories: as such they do not form a homogenous group. The type of problems that they encounter are many and varied, ranging from legal to personal, including sexual, problems. The nature of the sexual problems they face are no different than those faced by non-users, although their drug use may cause or be part of the cause for such problems.

It was recognised that drug users were perceived as deviant in most countries and as such were often alienated from the services that were available to other people within those countries. As a result of this deviant label, many myths have developed about drug users which are then often portrayed in policy and campaigns concerning drug use. Stereotypical images of the drug user are presented in media and literature campaigns which reinforce the alienation that drug users feel. These images and myths are often taken on by the wider society, including those who are providers of services which could be of use to drug users.

With the advent of HIV has come the further stigmatisation of drug users as a group of people, as they have been identified as being at risk of infection through the sharing of injecting equipment. Drug users have also been identified as a "bridge" of infection to the "wider heterosexual community". Whilst these categories might have some legitimacy in the field of epidemiology, they fail to take into account the responsibility of all persons, irrespective of drug using status, to protect themselves from infection by engaging in safer sex practices. They may reflect a prejudiced view of drug users as a "threat" to the "general public", rather than a group of individuals entitled to services and information in the interests of their own well-being.

Specialist Drug Services

Specialist drug services have been established in most European countries, although the range and extent of such services varies significantly, particularly in Eastern and Southern Europe. Specialist drug services were established to offer people with drug problems provision to overcome their problems. The prevailing philosophy among these services, pre-HIV, was to enable the drug user to cease taking drugs. They offered a range of provision including advice, counselling, residential rehabilitation and medical services. Some included legal and advocacy services in their provision.

The advent of HIV has led to a reassessment of the services needed to help drug users, especially those that have not traditionally attended services. The major change in provision was the introduction of access to clean injecting equipment to those who injected. In recognition of the fact that drug users were also sexual human beings, many agencies also included the availability of condoms and literature concerning safer sex. Drug agencies also recognised the importance of taking their services out to the user rather than rely on them coming into the agency. As a result of these changes agencies began to reach many more people.

The working group identified a range of problems that have emerged for workers in specialist agencies. Workers, having entered the drug field in order to help people with problems concerning their drug use, are now having to tackle a broader range of issues including changes in approach to their work.

Many drug workers find it difficult to discuss sexual matters with their clients. This is often due to a lack of confidence in their own abilities and a fear of entering into discussions which they may find embarrassing or difficult to deal with. Drug users may reinforce this behaviour on the part of workers, and seek to avoid the topic of sex if they have come to the agency for help with their drug use. Accordingly, most participants recognised that it was easier to help drug users to change their injecting drug habits than their sexual practices. It was also noted that the user's own denial of risk from sexual transmission would often be shared by his or her partner(s).

A second major change is the effect on drug workers of having to work with feelings of loss and change, and increasingly bereavement, with their clients. Whilst there has always been some element of this in drug work, it has significantly increased with the advent of HIV.

As a result of these changes, many workers feel inadequately supported and poorly equipped to carry out their work. They fear that if they reveal these anxieties to their managers they will be considered inefficient and lacking as workers, with the possibility of being disciplined. It was the clear view of the group that there was a lack of support structures available to deal with these needs. As a result of this, participants identified a noticeable increase in the burn-out rate amongst drug workers in their respective countries.

Training for Workers

It was recognised that the people who look after drug users as regards HIV are often different to those who look after them in terms of their drug use. Participants felt that by using a training needs analysis approach it would be possible to identify the different needs of these two groups and those areas that they had in common. Having identified these needs it will be essential to offer some joint training in order to capitalise on the range of skills and expertise within the workforce, and to encourage greater cooperation among disciplines. It is also important to train a range of people within an organisation, including management, if the work is to be effective and sustained.

Training was offered a low priority within the structures in which many participants operated, and this limited access to courses for both workers and organisations. Where training was provided, there was a further problem in that it could be perceived by some managers of services as the answer to all their problems, with the result that it was devalued later when the problems still remained. Yet the nature of these problems was more to do with organisational and managerial issues than to do with skills development concerning HIV. A properly constructed training needs analysis would enable many of these problems to be overcome, particularly if it was built into the common practice of the organisation as an employer.

Materials Concerning Drug Users

Most countries have developed a range of materials relevant to drug users. These materials take different forms including leaflets, comics and posters. They include information on how to avoid infection and/or transmission of HIV via drug use as well as sexual activity. Those that seemed to work best contained non-judgemental information concerning drug use, presented in language that was easy to understand. Those that were least successful contained stereotyped images of drug users, and based their information on negative reinforcement concerning the dangers of drug use.

Some concern was expressed over the use of comics particularly as regards the language and imagery used to describe sex. It was felt that there was a danger of falling into the trap of producing materials that could be seen as pornographic, or otherwise unappealing to women, rather than educative and informative. It was suggested that people should look at ways of using more traditional forms of art and take into account the sensitivities of all those who might have access to the materials. Involving drug users themselves in the development of materials was identified as one of the main ways to ensure their relevance. Effective targeting of materials was also seen as crucial in order to enable people to identify with the messages conveyed. Targeting needs to take into account the social class, ethnicity, gender, sexual orientation and literacy of the audience addressed. There also need to be specific materials for prison populations, recognising the situation in which they are located.

Non-Specialist Drug Services

Drug users do not rely exclusively upon specialist drug services. There are times when they need access to the full range of social care and medical provision. There was concern that drug users often receive poor treatment from non-specialist services and the main reason for this seems to lie within the stereotyping of drug users as a result of the myths that have been created about them. Drug users have found that some services are not accessible and are too rigid in their approach. This concern was particularly marked in relation to primary health care facilities, to which access is essential if drug users are to maintain their health.

It was felt that, given the skills and expertise in issues related to sex and sexuality available outside the drugs field, it was vital to encourage non-specialist services to work with drug users. For this to occur, specific training programmes need to be developed to address the problems that non-specialist workers may have regarding drug use.

Recommendations

The workshop ended by formulating the following recommendations, which the participants believed would aid development in addressing the sexual health needs of drug users:

1. Drug users must be recognised as sexual beings, representing the full range of human sexual experience, and should be afforded the same opportunities as the population as a whole to gain sexual health.

2. The war on drugs is a war on drug users and, as such, should end as it legitimises the alienation of drug users from the communities in which they live, thus inhibiting the effectiveness of health promotion, harm minimisation and HIV prevention strategies.

3. People who work with drug users require access to appropriate support and training in order to address sexual health issues. This should be an integral part of the service strategy and development. Training should provide balanced coverage of theoretical, attitudinal and emotional issues and practical skills.

4. Support must be provided to allow workers an opportunity to address the emotional impact of the work, in confidence, and this should not be linked to supervision concerning performance or discipline.

16

Condom Power: Roll on Responsibility

Background paper and report by Renée Aroney (author of background paper), Kobler Centre and John Hunter Clinic, Riverside Health Authority, London, with Margaret Jones (chairperson), Brook Advisory Centres, London

Other members of the group were:

Caroline Akehurst	*UK*
Kristina Bird	*UK*
Derek Bodell	*UK*
William Darrow	*USA*
Octavia Graur	*Romania*
Paul Hayton	*UK*
Ceri Hutton	*UK*
Lasse Kannas	*Finland*
Kurt Krikler	*Austria*
Krista Lewis	*UK*
Emmanuel Rusch	*France*
Roger Short	*Australia*
Brenda Spencer	*France*
Roger Staub	*Switzerland*
Stefan Thoelen	*Belgium*
Anita Weston	*UK*

Introduction

The condoms promotion working group was greatly disappointed that condoms were not supplied with each delegate's pack at the Promoting Sexual Health Workshop, as they were at the First International Workshop. One of the first principles of health promotion is to provide a positive role model. This can be achieved by providing condoms in delegates' packs at all future sexual health conferences, not necessarily for use at the conference, but as a symbol of commitment to promotion of use and to ensure that the theme of safer sex and prevention is placed high on the list of priorities by both organizers and delegates.

As health professionals and health educators we need to acknowledge that we are a vital and intrinsic body of key communicators in spreading the message of safer sex. All health professionals need to explore their own feelings, reservations and competence in promoting the use of condoms. Training and education of the educators is required in order for the condom to become a normal, routine and accepted part of health promotion and of sexual expression.

The major thrust of global AIDS prevention programmes is the promotion of condoms. We need to eroticize the condom, make it cool and trendy and perpetually fashionable to use. We must identify the needs of people for whom information, access, income, belief systems, social and cultural issues inhibit the use of condoms, and part of this process involves debunking the myths about condoms, HIV/AIDS and other STDs.

In contrast to AIDS programmes, STD control programmes have traditionally adopted the "medical model" — based on screening, diagnosis and treatment in conjunction with counselling and contact-tracing, rather than primary prevention. However, with growing alarm over the incidence of STDs, particularly HIV, increasing emphasis has been placed on primary prevention by promoting the use of condoms. Research has shown that, if used consistently and correctly, condoms are effective in preventing the transmission and acquisition of most STDs through vaginal and/or anal intercourse[1]. Condoms are also a reliable method of contraception without any of the side effects that the oral contraceptive and intra-uterine devices can have. They do not provide a 100% guarantee of safety, since they can and do break, but are the best protection available. However, it has been suggested that over-emphasis on contraception may obscure the fact that condoms also prevent the spread of STDs.

STDs such as syphilis and gonorrhoea have been declining in industrialised countries, especially amongst gay men, who first took up safer sex in the light of their perceived risk of HIV. Statistics now show a reversal of this original decline. The incidence of STDs such as genital warts, herpes simplex and chlamydia remains very high and studies show that men and women are still unaware that:

(a)   Chlamydia in women is usually asymptomatic in the early stages but if left untreated can lead to PID and possibly infertility;

(b)   The genital wart virus has been linked with cervical cancer;

(c)   The presence of STDs and genital ulceration can act as co-factors in enhancing the transmission of HIV[2].

Condom use may increase if people realise the high risks of contracting these other STDs. Mounting campaigns against chlamydia and gonorrhoea may be one way of encouraging condom use. Hence key facts about other STDs should be incorporated in condom promotion campaigns, without employing scare tactics (which are not successful in achieving behaviour changes[3]).

Safer sex is about having the confidence and conviction to say *no* to unwanted sex or unprotected sex. Negotiation of safer sex is complex and is the key area to focus on. Sexual partners, particularly women, need encouragement to feel confident to discuss safer sex and there is a need to promote the view that condom use and safer sex is the responsibility of both partners.

The task is to increase the number of people using condoms; to increase the frequency of their use; to increase correct usage; and particularly to ensure their use among people engaging in high risk practices for HIV and other STDs.

Marketing History of the Condom

Condom promotion campaigns can have multifaceted goals and people may use condoms for one or more of these reasons: to reduce the incidence of HIV and other STDs; to prevent unwanted pregnancy; and to reduce cervical cell abnormalities. Before the introduction of the oral contraceptive, the condom was the most popular method of birth control but by the mid-seventies the pill had become the most widely used method. Currently young people tend to use the most easily available method – ie. the condom – and then change to the oral contraceptive as relationships stabilise.

Availability of condoms is one of their main perceived advantages: no prescription is required (except in the Republic of Ireland); medical supervision is unnecessary; and to many they appear quite easy to use. However, putting on a condom is not as easy as putting on a pair of socks – there are steps which need to be taken to maximise its effectiveness. Also, putting on a pair of socks of does not demand self-esteem and self-confidence.

Research has shown that the main motivational and behavioural obstacles to the use and acceptability of condoms include:

1.   Belief that one is not personally at risk for HIV and other STDs;
2.   Embarrassment about buying condoms;
3.   Difficulty in raising the subject with one's partner;
4.   Belief that condoms reduce sexual pleasure;
5.   Uncertainties about effectiveness and reliability;
6.   Objection to the interruption of sex[4].

Other practical obstacles include lack of availability, lack of information on how to use condoms, religious barriers and other stigmas associated with using condoms eg. that they used to be promoted in military populations for servicemen having sex with prostitutes and in many countries are associated in people's minds with illicit or extramarital sex, prostitution and promiscuity. The challenge for condom promotion is to acknowledge that condoms do prevent STDs and promote them positively as a way whereby individuals can take responsibility for their own sexual health.

The health action model[5] illustrates and summarises all the factors that need to be taken into account when planning a condom promotion campaign, for all target groups, whether in a London Health Authority, a village in Uganda or at European level.

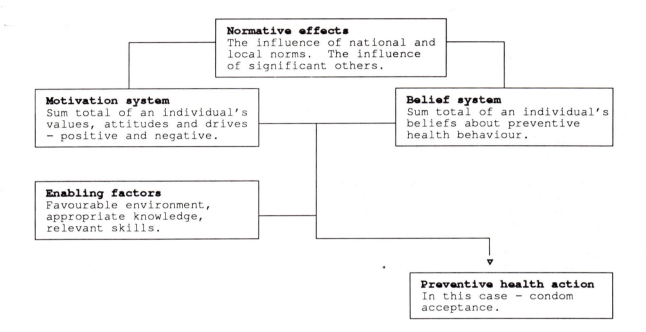

In reviewing the literature on condom promotion campaigns, one finds that it largely focusses on studies assessing the values of specific target groups towards condoms rather than evaluating campaigns that have actually taken place. Perhaps this reflects the fact that concerned health workers undertaking campaigns (not government mass media campaigns) lack resources and time fully to document and write up their work.

Target Audience

Condom promotion strategies range from targetting the general public through TV, radio and cinema advertisements to specific one-to-one safer sex counselling for STD clinic attenders requesting an HIV test, or the free distribution of condoms to clients attending needle exchange units and family planning clinics.

It is important to prioritise and target those individuals engaging in high risk activities for HIV and other STDs for financial and epidemiological reasons, as protection tends to be less common among those at the greatest risk of contracting HIV. The more precisely the programme is targetted the more likely it is to hit this real audience and the individual needs, wants and motivations of the specific target audience. Poorly targetted programmes are difficult to evaluate and may give mixed messages.

Regardless of how precisely targetting occurs, specific audiences are likely to overlap. For example a young heterosexual person still at school, who may also use drugs or be a short term client in social services care, could receive messages about condoms as part of a school health education programme, through staff at his or her care unit, through needle exchange workers or via the newspapers and TV, as well as from his/her peers. The basis of targetting should be effective planning and delivery of programmes, rather than labelling and directing of

...he emphasis should continue to be behaviour which puts people at risk rather than groups of people ...at risk.

Other working groups at this conference are looking at specific target groups and sexual health and the issue of condom promotion should be on the agenda for each and every group. The following are some groups that we believe need special attention:

- *Young People*

A recent study conducted by the University of Exeter found that 53% of school pupils between the ages of 16 and 17 had more than three sexual partners. Over half of this number had not used a condom during intercourse. Young people have the knowledge about risks of HIV infection, but need more skills and motivation to use condoms. A study from the University of Strathclyde found that less than 33% of 16-24 year olds use condoms regularly, despite knowing that they reduce the risk of HIV transmission. It was found they saw condoms as unattractive and problematic and safer sex difficult. A study from New York city showed adolescents were more inclined to use condoms if they believed their friends were doing so. Thus condom use amongst young people is associated with peer variables including peer acceptability, and one's own perceived ability. Many young people believe it is safe to have sex without a condom or any form of contraception during the female partner's period because "she won't get pregnant", and may not realise that this is a prime time for HIV to be transmitted through infected menstrual blood.

- *Injecting Drug Users*

In the USA it has been found that two thirds of the cases of AIDS in heterosexuals were due to HIV infection acquired from sexual partners who were injecting drug users[6]. The transmission rate depends on the extent of equipment sharing and of unsafe sex[7]. A study in North London showed that whilst the majority of drug users had adopted safer drug using practices, only 31% of injecting drug users were practising safer sex. Drug dependency units and needle exchange schemes play a key role in providing the resources and support for sexual and drug taking risk reduction and act as a source of referral to other agencies.

- *Men who have sex with men*

The gay community first heeded the warnings about HIV and developed safer sex practices. Existing structures of an established community assisted in spreading the safer sex/condom message through gay bars, saunas and meeting places, eg a gay bar in Paris uses the Australian Condom Man poster *"Don't be shame be game use condoms"*. While condom use is reported to have greatly increased among gay and bisexual men as a result of the AIDS epidemic, it is important to know about the variables influencing lack of use. These have been cited as impairment of pleasure, unavailability at time of intercourse and influence of drugs and alcohol. Prevention programmes that concentrate solely on the dangers of unprotected anal intercourse may not adequately address other factors such as improper use, inadequate or inappropriate lubrication, or belief that one is safe in a monogamous relationship. For example, on many occasions gay men have requested convenient sized sachets of lubricants.

Ross[8], in Australia, identified further variables associated with lack of change to safer sex amongst gay and bisexual men – such as depression and psychological maladjustment, which may suggest that psychological support is needed. Other factors include social skills, personality characteristics and economic circumstances. Some gay men who have been practising safer sex for many years are now returning to less safe behaviour and this may be more common among HIV seropositive men, raising concerns about the possible risks of repeated exposure to HIV in accelerating progression to AIDS. Among studies reported at the VIth International Conference on AIDS in San Francisco were reports from England that gay men under the age of 21 (the legal age of consent for male homosexual acts) were having more risky sex than their elders, reflecting lack of access to health education resulting from legal restrictions and absence of non-judgemental sex education in schools; and from Finland that from 1983-9, with increasing personal counselling and growing media coverage, there had been increased condom use during anal sex but not for oral sex.

It is important for health professionals to be positive in their recommendations for safer sex and to acknowledge that safer sex messages can at times be confusing, eg recommendations to use condoms during oral sex even though the risk of HIV transmission is low or that in anal intercourse even with a condom the penis should be withdrawn prior to ejaculation.

• *Women*

In the booklet "Don't Die of Ignorance — I nearly died of embarrassment"[9] the authors discuss a UK TV ad which showed a young woman trying to negotiate safer sex with a male partner in which the male voice-over comments "and she's too embarrassed to ask him to use a condom....wouldn't it have been easier to talk about it earlier?" They argue that embarrassment about using condoms and difficulty in negotiating their use is far more complex than merely bad timing.

The social, sexual and financial insecurity which exists between men and women in most societies gives rise to many issues for women in negotiating safer sex with men. A woman's ability to introduce condom use to her male partner demands pre-existing enabling conditions such as:

- Relative sexual equality between men and women;
- A possibility for acknowledging other sex partners without seriously threatening the relationship;
- The existence of options other than motherhood to define self-identity or self-esteem for women.

Further issues are that a woman who suggests using a condom may be perceived as deviating from the cultural norm by not being passive and that a woman who buys or carries condoms may risk her reputation and be perceived as "a slut". There is also a perception amongst women that men find condoms uncomfortable which makes women reticent to suggest or insist on their use. We need to find ways of empowering women to be more assertive in sexual relationships in order to promote sexual safety.

Prostitutes

Studies have shown that sex workers are more likely to wear condoms with commercials clients than with their partners, and this presents a particular challenge for health promotion.

Minority Ethnic Groups

More research is needed to investigate how specific cultural norms affect sexual decision-making. It is very difficult for an individual to use condoms if this practice is not regarded as appropriate in his/her community. In this situation one of the goals of the programme could be to change the community position on condom use. In New York it was found that condom promotion campaigns aimed at Hispanics needed to take into account the cultural discomfort of talking about sex in mixed sex groups and use themes that are powerful in Latino culture, such as safe-guarding fertility and protecting one's family.

Health Promotion Experience

Throughout the world, in industrialised and developing countries, some very innovative and imaginative condom promotion campaigns have been promoted through schools, family planning and STD clinics, voluntary organisations, the media, by condom manufacturers, pop and sporting stars, fashion designers and workers in the sex industry. Here is a taste of the international smorgasbord of interventions and campaigns that have taken place, are currently taking place or are planned:-

- *6 tips for hard cocks*, a pamphlet produced by the AIDS Council of New South Wales explicitly showing the correct steps to putting on a condom, aimed at gay and bisexual men with photos of erect penises.

- The safer sex condom guide for men and women produced by the Gay Men's Health Crisis in New York City, again illustrating correct condom usage with photos of different erect penises.
- Since 1985 all STD clinics in New South Wales have offered free condoms to clients attending for check-ups — a condom for each visit.

- Safer Sex Outreach Teams/Condom Squads are becoming very popular throughout the world, eg for World AIDS Day 1990 staff at a London clinic distributed 10,000 free condoms sellotaped to a condom guide to both members of the general public and to staff at the hospital. The previous year 3000 condoms had been distributed at Covent Garden — but many were rendered ineffective by stapling to a leaflet.

- In Sydney the Super Secret Society of Simply Stunning Safe Sex Sluts (volunteers from AIDS Council of New South Wales) distribute free condoms and sachets of lubricant regularly at most major community events such as World AIDS Day, Mardi Gras, Opera in the Park. At the 1987 Montreux Jazz Festival in Switzerland special condom holders with condoms were distributed.

- In Finland in 1990 the government mailed a 16 page sex education magazine called "SEXTIIN" to all 16 year olds with a condom enclosed.

- Local health authorities in London are now advertising for "condom project workers" where the remit is to improve the availability and accessibility of condoms to sexually active people.

- In Amsterdam an extremely exciting condom shop opened in 1987, where the proprietors "wanted to do away with the taboo associated with the sale of condoms". The shop is called the "Condomerie" (a pun on the German Konditerie for cakes) and is suitable for the whole family to browse in. Such a shop greatly reduces the stigma and embarrassment surrounding condoms.

- World AIDS Day 1990 saw the video and musical releases of Red, Hot and Blue around the world, with popular stars such as Neneh Cherry, Annie Lennox and Deborah Harry singing to raise awareness about safer sex, and reduce the stigma surrounding HIV and AIDS.

- In her 1990 world tour Madonna said in her concerts "Don't be silly, put a condom on your willy".

- A small item in the Lancet on September 22 1990 advertised the new plastic condom demonstrator put out by Durex, which stimulated a competing company to also produce one. The demonstrator is designed for family planning clinics, general practices, schools and health promotion departments. Some places use dildoes, the Brook Advisory Centres (for young people) use a lifelike penile model, which some may find threatening, while others use plastic bananas which are non-threatening and can make the client smile.

- An Australian study[10] looked at attitudes among young multi-partner heterosexuals and their implications for design of condom promotion campaigns. It suggested campaigns should: acknowledge the embarrassment of suggesting condom use and show that this fear is groundless; and provide more socially acceptable or less awkward ways of naming or mentioning condoms — using brand names, euphemisms or humour. For example a New Zealand campaign called condoms parachutes — as in "Would you like to come parachuting with me?" It is planned in South Australia to call condoms "nightcaps" — as in "Would you like to come back to my place for a night cap?" Brand name advertising gives the potential consumer a name to ask for.

- The Hot Rubber and Stop AIDS Campaigns in Switzerland have been extremely successful, using billboard posters portraying condoms in effective ways such as the setting sun (a large condom) going down over an idyllic sea setting. All Migros supermarkets in Switzerland sell condoms and lubricant.

- A recent Australian health promotion campaign aimed at gay men which says *"You'll never forget the feeling of safe sex"* is attempting to address the attitude that condom use reduces sexual pleasure/sensation. There is no denying the loss of sensation, but this needs to be counter-balanced against freedom from worry about STDs and HIV.

- Another Australian campaign included a sticker saying *"Tell him if it's not on, it's not on"*. This slogan enhances the assertive role a woman or man can play in wanting protected intercourse. Another campaign, against chlamydia, shows male and female pairs of eyes with the caption *"Gaze into these eyes and practise saying 'Sure I'll use a condom'."* Such campaigns elevate the community's awareness about negotiating safer sex.

- In Japan, where condom use is greater than anywhere else in the world (in 1986 45% of couples used condoms for contraception), a novel sales approach is for manufacturers to hire door-to-door condom saleswomen. Housewives are the target audience while husbands are at work and children at school. Condom popularity in Japan is due partly to the fact that oral contraception is illegal and IUDs expensive. Japan has novelty musical condoms — together with brand names such as *"Here come the Giants"* and *"Almighty"*. (It is important that if condom sizes become available these should not be small, medium and large, but "large", "extra large" and "oh my God".)

- In The Netherlands knowledge that condoms prevent HIV transmission is high. In October 1987 a campaign to make condoms more socially acceptable was launched, using 30 well known Dutch people, saying that they use "them". Free condoms in attractive packaging were distributed along with posters and cinema advertisements. The campaign was aimed in stages at the general public as well as targetting specific audiences such as adolescents.

- In the UK the latest AIDS campaign is directed at every sexually active person. TV ads feature six anonymous personal testimonies from HIV positive people — three heterosexual women, two gay men (the first time gay men have been acknowledged in the government campaign) and one heterosexual man. The ads received a mixed reaction for being too subtle about condom use and employing scare tactics. Another cinema ad intended to decrease embarrassment and uncertainty about condom use features a woman named Mrs Dawson at work in a condom factory — ending with a slogan *"Keep Mrs Dawson busy, use a condom"*.

- The best known effort to promote condoms in a developing country, prior to the recognition of HIV, was that of the Population and Community Development Association of Thailand. As a result of the campaign the condom became a household word. Condoms were put on display everywhere, blown up into balloons, etc.

- It is difficult to promote condoms in developing countries due to varying cultural norms and perceptions of the male's role in the family planning. In Egypt a mass media campaign promoting a brand of condoms ran into censorship problems because it emphasized family planning as a joint responsibility and displayed a man and woman with wedding rings holding a pack of condoms. The censors wanted the removal of the woman's hand, thus reinforcing the man's powerful role of taking full responsibility.

- Roger Short developed a peer group AIDS educational programme aimed at medical students over a two year period at Monash University.

Building Healthy Public Policy

In order to promote condoms it is important to have the framework of a sexual health policy to work within: such a policy framework would include making a commitment to sexual health education in schools, and enabling condoms to be normalised and their use made an expression of healthy lifestyle, thus converting the idea of disease into one of prevention. An international model sexual health policy should be developed which recognises the right of all people to express their sexuality positively in a fulfilling and satisfying way without abusing the rights of others. This policy should set out the inalienable right of young people to become sexually aware and to prevent unplanned pregnancies, HIV and other STDs transmission; it should be non-judgemental and provide clear and accurate information from educators experienced and trained in this field. Sexual health education in schools should begin at primary level and condoms should be handled and discussed in schools by pupils of primary school age. All teacher training should contain input on safer sex and condoms. Key teachers in each school should be nominated for training in this area.

It is important that condoms have government and health department endorsement through advertising. The health department stands for impartiality and objectivity and can promote the concept of condoms as a healthy product rather than by brand. Health departments are more likely to be believed than manufacturers when they say that condoms help prevent STDs including HIV and are an effective method of birth control. Effective policy implementation may require government processes to be simplified. For instance, in the UK the Department of Health currently needs to work with the Department of Education and Science on issues such as safer sex education in school, the Department of Environment about local authority health issues, the Home Office on prisons, the Department of Trade about standards and monopolies in the condom market, and the Department of Employment on workplace issues.

Official health promotion should include campaigns on STDs other than HIV, such as chlamydia and PID prevention campaigns endorsing the use of condoms. Health authorities in the UK are formulating condom policies and appointing condom project workers — this should happen on an international scale.

In the UK there is no production standard for condoms for anal intercourse, and such a standard needs to be introduced as at present it is impossible to know which brands are reliable for anal use. Gay men need access to this information as do heterosexuals if they are having anal intercourse. In the UK a study showed that 3.5% of men and 4.5% of women had experienced anal sex by the age of 18[11]. Under the existing standard condoms must conform to both lower and upper thickness limits. The upper limit should be removed so that thicker condoms in gay outlets can be covered by an international standard.

It is for governments to ensure that the price of condoms remains reasonable and that they meet high standards of quality. However, studies show that cost is not always a major problem – condoms are cheaper than cigarettes. Throughout the world much money is set aside for medical research into HIV and AIDS – should a percentage be set aside to provide *free* condoms for sexually active people to whom cost may be an issue? Government funding should support community-based and outreach services to those who are most at risk. Frontline health settings such as STD clinics, young people's contraceptive services and drug agencies should provide a wide variety of condoms, spermicide and lubricants and dental dams to their clients who may not have sufficient money, motivation and confidence to purchase condoms. STD clinics need increased funding as they see individuals at high risk for STDs and AIDS and large numbers of people having unsafe sex, as do family planning clinics which see many people potentially at risk. In the UK it has been suggested that general practitioners should also supply condoms freely to patients but funding for this additional cost to regional health authorities has not yet been agreed.

There are many other measures which could be taken:

- Governments could endorse a policy whereby supermarkets, shopping centres and public transport services designate community service areas in their premises for health workers to promote condoms in National Condom Week or on World AIDS Day, and encourage such places to provide poster space for condom advertisements.

- There could be a legally enforced minimum number of condom vending machines in commercial, institutional and work-place settings in each health authority.

- An audit of condom sales should be officially conducted, as in the USA where 2% of drug stores are involved in a regular condom audit.

- Governments could provide tax incentives to film makers who mention condoms in their movies.

The group believed that more funding should be directed to basic research on the properties of condoms, as lack of information hampers condom promotion strategies. The World Health Organisation and the European Medical Research Council should be funded to set up a condom research and information centre to examine method and user failure/success rates of condoms in preventing unplanned pregnancy, transmission of HIV and other STDs and also to investigate the user failure/success rates in age-related, behavioural and socio-economic contexts. More research is needed into the efficacy of spermicides and dental dams and development of female barrier methods to prevent HIV and STD transmission.

Creating Supportive Environments

Availability and accessibility are key factors influencing condom use. We need to acknowledge that embarrassment is a key factor in the purchasing of condoms — to overcome this vending machines should be placed in discreet locations such as toilet cubicles in meeting places such as discos, clubs, hotels, cinemas, railway stations, theatres, take away food outlets and tertiary education institutions. According to the London Rubber Company modern designs are making condom vending machines more popular, eg the Durex dual vending machine, which stocks a choice of condom brands or of one brand and a tampon, is popular in the UK and Holland. Mail order is also becoming popular and overcomes the embarrassment factor.

Some pharmacies still need to be encouraged to have condoms on open display. Many products vie for the position next to the cash register in commercial outlets such as pharmacies and supermarkets — priority should be given to condoms together with lubricants.

In the UK there has been drop in the percentage of condoms obtained from family planning clinics due to cuts in these services. Less than half of all men know that condoms are available free of charge for them at such clinics.

It is very difficult for an individual to use condoms if the practice is not regarded as appropriate in his/her community — there is a need to change community attitudes to condoms. They should be available in schools where students should have access to experiential workshops on condoms and where correct condom use should be demonstrated by teachers.

International/European Condom Logo

Both the last workshop and this working group believed a European logo for condoms should be developed for display at the entrance to all premises where condoms are on sale, along the lines of the international credit card signs. Local authorities and councils could also display the sign on the boundary of their areas, to indicate one is entering a zone where the use of condoms is endorsed. In Australia sex workers have devised a safe house scheme along these lines, where a yellow triangle is displayed at the entrance of establishments where managers make it a house rule that condoms are used for all acts of intercourse and oral sex. Clients refusing condoms are refused service. Such measures provide a supportive environment for the workers. There are benefits all around since the clientele are educated to expect condom use as the norm and the establishment gains an enhanced reputation as a low risk establishment.

Women's Rights

Community awareness of sexual inequality needs to be raised and the social, legal and cultural conditions that allow these inequalities to persist need to be removed so that women become able to carry and introduce the use of condoms without being made to feel "easy" or labelled a "slut".

Condom Manufacturers

Manufacturers can have a role in creating supportive environments – the London Rubber Company aims to remove embarrassment surrounding the purchase and use of condoms; to correct false negative associations that people have about condoms; and to communicate safer sex in an understandable way.

The group felt that manufacturers need to develop more marketing initiatives and bolder advertising campaigns, and diversify their product ranges. They should play a much larger role in making condoms "hip" and more acceptable. They need to address consumer complaints about taste, smell, sensation and packaging, be more daring in these areas, and advertise/provide sachets of water-based lubricants with each condom rather than the often cumbersome large tubes that are now available. Condoms should be included in airline packs, women's toiletry packs, etc.

Image

Condoms need to be relevant to people's life-style. Young people are not attracted to condoms by packaging and advertising better-suited to the staid family planning consumer or to the customer looking for a sex aid "ribbed for her pleasure". Gay men are unlikely to buy a packet of condoms with a picture of a man and a woman on the front — manufacturers should look at new ways of marketing their product to attract new consumer groups. For example, recently Durex repackaged their Safe Play condoms in black packets with flip top lids like cigarette packs (somewhat ironically, for such a healthy product) to make them more appealing to young people.

Mass media advertising makes condoms acceptable. Health workers and teachers promoting condoms to individuals and small groups are like a condom team going into battle. Their job is made much easier by improved image and community acceptance, which can be effectively assisted by mass media advertising.

Such advertising campaigns need to address:

• Reducing consumer embarrassment over buying condoms;

• Giving positive role models for negotiating safer sex for men and women;

• The need for men to take responsibility for birth control and disease prevention, and promotion of the idea that women will be impressed by such initiative.

Educating health workers and teachers

For any condom campaign to succeed, health workers need to feel positive, confident and comfortable promoting condoms. It is important that training is provided to frontline workers such as STD and family planning physicians, GPs, nurses and counsellors in these settings and to drug workers. Teachers need in-service training in aspects of sexuality to enable them to discuss sexual health issues and the prevention of HIV and STD transmission with their pupils.

Strengthening Community Action

Condom outreach programmes have varied from mobile vans distributing free condoms, to colourful safer sex stalls in public places, to people dressing up as condoms in street theatre. Positive-minded health workers endorsing the use of condoms in this way provide positive role models.

People who shape community opinion, pop, sport and film stars, need to speak out regularly in support of condoms. There should be local condom resource centres, 24 hour free condom recorded information lines and National Condom Weeks. A rap song on the correct 10 steps to put on a condom would do a lot to promote condom use and could become top of the pops. Local condom campaigns need to be part of the community – youth clubs, churches, professional and trade associations, community organisations such as neighbourhoods, community groups and clubs, and places of local entertainment could all be involved.

Developing Personal Skills

Personal skills which need to be developed within condom campaigns include correct and consistent use and how to negotiate in sexual encounters. The majority of skills training takes place on a one-to-one basis between counsellor and client or in small group discussions, with mass media campaigns enhancing this work. Peer education for adolescents is an important intervention to explore.

Some health workers have reservations about broaching the subject of condoms with their clients. One disadvantage of condoms is that they have to be thought about at the time of intercourse and young people in particular may be thought to lack sufficient self-confidence. However, it is not an insult to advise clients on how they can prevent disease and unwanted pregnancy. Word-of-mouth information to clients is important to show that condom use is recommended and held in high regard by health professionals. It is also important for the counsellor to show that they understand the reservations the client might have, while still projecting a positive image of condoms. For example if a client complains that condoms cause a loss of sensation then the counsellor should acknowledge that there may be a slight loss of sensation, but also stress the benefits such as freedom from worry about STDs or that the loss of sensation may help them to prolong intercourse. Clients who are reluctant to use condoms because of past negative experiences should be reassured that condom design and safety have improved.

A UK study surveying contraceptive practices and reasons for contraceptive failure among women attending for abortion counselling and referral noted a rise among young women requesting termination of pregnancy which has been linked to incorrect condom use[12]. Reported problems such as condoms breaking or slipping off indicate the need for client education about correct condom use. Thus first timers at clinics and other agencies or those who are not confident about using condoms should be given demonstrations on how to use a condom correctly and encouragement to practice.

What to tell clients/pupils/students

It is important to encourage everyone to carry condoms with them at all times, regardless of whether they are expecting to have sex or not. Carrying condoms does not mean a person is "easy" or promiscuous. It means they are smart and always prepared like the boy scouts. Clients should be encouraged to think about condom use before they reach the bedroom and to think that protection from STDs is as important as contraception. The very nicest person can have an STD and prevention is better than cure (and for AIDS there is no cure). Many potential lovers may be unaware of any infection, especially those with long incubation periods such as AIDS, wart virus and herpes, so asking about sexual history is no protection. It is better to take responsibility for yourself by using condoms. In the context of a relationship where condoms are not used, the couple should be encouraged to agree to use condoms if either of them has sex outside the relationship or has had previous relationships. For young people in their first relationship this means exploring with them the possibility of other future relationships. The key message is:

Safer sex is 100% your responsibility and 100% your partner's – it's not 50/50

Condom check list

Health workers and teachers should emphasise that correct use can minimise the possibility of condom breakage and other sources of failure. Male clients can be encouraged *to familiarise themselves with condoms by wearing one while masturbating* — and female clients to take the condom out of the packet to feel it, to blow it up, etc.

The 10 steps to using a condom are:

1. Check the expiry date and ensure that the condoms conform with the country's standard.

2. Tear the packet open and squeeze condom out like toothpaste.

3. Make sure that rings and fingernails don't snag the condom.

4. Put the condom onto the erect penis before any type of penetration has taken place.

5. Squeeze the teat of the condom between thumb and index finger.

6. Place the rolled up condom on the glans having first drawn back the foreskin.

7. Roll the condom on the erect penis and make sure that it goes all the way down to the base of the penis. Be aware that it should unroll easily.

8. Use additional water-based lubricants and spermicide if necessary. Some men like to squeeze some lubricant into the teat of the condom before they put it on.

9. Withdraw after ejaculation while the penis is still stiff and hold the condom at the base of the penis during withdrawal.

10. Dispose of the condom in the garbage rather than the toilet. (Recognise that young people may wish to flush it down the toilet for fear of discovery.)

People who suffer from skin irritation from condoms are recommended to experiment with different brands which may not contain spermicide or brands intended for people with allergies. If a condom breaks it is recommended that the penis is withdrawn immediately. The packet and remaining condoms should be kept and the incident reported to the manufacturer. Where condoms are used for contraception there is the option of taking emergency "post-coital" contraception within 72 hours.

The ideal instruction leaflet should be small and pictorial to minimise problems of language and illiteracy. It should offer suggestions on how to introduce condom use to a partner, and include facts about STDs and HIV — where to get help and advice (eg 24 hour information line).

Suggesting what to say to a sexual partner

What is appropriate depends a lot on personal style. Clients should be encouraged to "be themselves" unless this has proved unsuccessful in the past. Counsellors should offer some ideas to clients, ie condom "come on" lines:

> "No condom, no sex."
> "I always use condoms."
> "I'll show you — let me put it on with my mouth."
> "I'm not on the pill so let's use these." (Hold up condoms).
> "We can use my condoms if you haven't got any."
> "Don't worry — I'll put it on nicely for you."
> "Is a condom OK with you?"
> "If you can't be bothered to get the condoms — that's OK — we'll just play — we won't go all the way this time."

These suggestions may assist the client to get over their embarrassment surrounding condoms. For clients who say that condoms are passion killers or disrupt the flow of sex, one can suggest laying the condoms our ready, out of their packs, to be picked up and put on.

Audio-visual material in waiting rooms can show role plays of negotiating condom use with a partner. Audio-visual material aimed at specific target audiences can be useful, eg the Australian *"Work safe – play safe"* video for sex workers, which covers questions such as "How do you put on a condom properly?" and "What is safer sex?" or the American Gay Men's Health Crisis video for gay men on safer sex, showing explicitly how to use condoms and dental dams, with no voice-overs, just music and action on the screen. Videos and materials/leaflets need to be produced in many languages to reach those whose main language is not the national one. Videos for specific ethnic groups can take into account the customs and attitudes of these groups and can be shown in community-based settings specific to the target audience on a one-to-one basis with a counsellor. The new Red Cross material *"Your choice or mine?"* provides over 50 role play situations for use with young people.

Some issues on which health workers need guidance to advise clients: lubricants, spermicide and dental dams

Condom supplies from key services are inadequate, but usually lubricants are not available at all. There is confusion in the community about the role and uses of lubricants and spermicide.

Condom promotion campaigns need to take into account the very important role of lubricants and spermicide. There has been conflicting information on the use of nonoxynol 9 following the VIth International Conference on AIDS in San Francisco, where it was reported that nonoxynol 9 is an irritant and should not be used. However this related to very heavy levels of use. People need to be educated about the benefits of spermicide and lubricants and wider availability of these products ensured along with condoms. The damaging effects of oil/petroleum-based lubricants on latex also need publicising. People in the community are hearing more about dental dams – there is a need to clarify their role and the advice we should be giving about their use.

Re-orienting Services

In STD and family planning clinics and drug agencies, prevention of STDs and HIV should form an essential part of every consultation. Clients of these agencies should be given the safer sex message on every visit – otherwise the professionals are failing in their duty. Condoms and leaflets should be available in toilets and waiting rooms. If free condoms are available they should be offered to everyone who attends the clinic, regardless of their reason for attending.

STD clinics in particular should become primary prevention sites where each person entering receives a safer sex message and kit, including condoms, lubrication and an information sheet on their use and strategies for negotiating safer sex. At present there is no guarantee that each person entering a clinic receives safer sex information so a stamp for clinic notes should be developed stating "safer sex information given". Clients requesting HIV testing provide an opportune time to discuss condoms and safer sex practices.

Family planning and abortion clinics should also re-orient services by raising issues of STD and HIV prevention and endorsing the use of condoms. Drug agencies deal with harm minimalisation/needle exchange and are broaching the subject of using condoms and safer sex. Alcohol and homelessness projects, probation, social services, education facilities, youth clubs and youth projects can all be used as places to increase condom awareness and venues where condoms are available. The role of prevention needs to be better recognised, and money for condom research is vital to provide a real weapon to prevent HIV transmission.

General practitioners in the general community can play a greater role in promoting safer sex — their waiting rooms could carry more posters about use of condoms against pregnancy and STDs. They could show videos and GPs and their nursing staff could give condom demonstrations and discuss difficulties of negotiating safer sex.

Final Recommendations

It was felt that there was insufficient time, unfortunately, to explore and make recommendations on all the issues that had been raised in the working group. The group was dismayed to discover that none of the recommendations from the condom working group at the previous workshop had been implemented. Therefore we have suggested to whom our recommendations should be addressed in the hope that the organizers of the workshop will take them up with the suggested authorities.

Our Group's recommendations are:

1. The Promoting Sexual Health Workshop sponsors should support a group to develop a model sexual health policy recognising the right of all people to express their sexuality positively in a fulfilling and satisfying way without abusing the rights of others. This policy should be relevant to all, but with particular reference to the inalienable right of young people to become sexually aware, to prevent unplanned pregnancies and HIV and other STDs transmission; it should be non-judgemental and allow recipients to receive clear and accurate information from educators experienced and trained in this field. Such a policy should include for all and in particular for young people:

    i) Easy and earlier access to condoms in youth settings and generally wider availability of condoms, eg not just in pharmacies, but supermarkets, tabacs, petrol stations, in places where people meet people, with more condom vending machines placed discreetly in areas such as toilet cubicles.

    ii) Recognition of the necessity for teaching practical skills in the correct use of condoms and lubricants. The feelings and reservations that professionals such as teachers, drug workers and general practitioners may have about their professional competence in promoting condoms need to be addressed — eg drug workers may see their role as dealing with harm minimization for safer drug use rather than also being safer sex educators.

    iii) Removal of all impediments to the access to information on condoms, particularly in educational settings.

2. We believe that lack of information hampers condom promotion strategies and recommend that the following questions should be examined by the World Health Organisation as well as the European Medical Research Councils (as it was felt that the EMRC had greater influence in Eastern Europe):

    i) To examine the efficacy of methods and user failure/success rates for using condoms in preventing:
       (a) unplanned pregnancy;
       (b) transmission of HIV;
       (c) transmission of other STDs.

    ii) To investigate the user failure/success rates in behavioural and socio-economic context.

    iii) To investigate the efficacy of and evaluate and devise new female barrier methods such as the female condom; spermicide; lubricants; condoms impregnated with spermicide and dental dams.

iv) To carry out a thorough condom literature review and make the resulting review widely available.

Thus we recommend that a *Condom Research and Information Centre* be established which would coordinate all this information from the following four WHO programmes, all of which have access to information and databases on condoms within their remit: the Global Programme on AIDS; the Maternal and Child Health programme; the family planning programme; the STDs programme: and that interim findings from this centre be published regularly in WHO newsletters.

3. We agree with the recommendations of the last condom working group which were primarily directed at the condom manufacturers. We wish to emphasise and reiterate the recommendation for development of a European standard for condoms which would be readily recognisable by a symbol which would appear on the condom packet and the outlets through which they are available. This symbol should be as recognisable as and placed beside Visa, Mastercard and American Express signs. We deplore the lack of marketing initiatives, advertising campaigns and diversification of product ranges by the condom manufacturers.

4. Organisers of all future sexual health conferences should place condoms in the delegates' document packs handed out on registration.

5. There should be professional development and training for all health professionals, including nurses, doctors and counsellors, teachers in schools, drugs workers, general practitioners, etc. on issues surrounding condoms such as the correct steps in their use, negotiating their use, and raising the topic of condom use and safer sex in any consultations on sexual health.

References

1. Conant M, Hardy D, Sernantiger J Spicer D, Levy J A. Condoms prevent transmission of AIDS-associated retrovirus. JAMA 1986; **255**: 1706.

2. Rowen D, Carne C. Heterosexual transmission of HIV. Int J STDs and AIDS 1990: 239-244.

3. Sherr L. Health education. AIDS Care 1989; **1(2)**: 188-192.

4. Wellings K. Position statement on condoms. AIDS Programme. London: Health Education Authority, 1989.

5. Tones B K. Past achievement and future success. *In:* Sutherland I (ed). Health education: perspectives and choices. London: Allen and Unwin, 1979.

6. Moss A R. AIDS and intravenous drug use: the real heterosexual epidemic. Br Med J 1987; **294**: 389-90.

7. Hart G J, Carvell A, Johnson A M, Feinmann C, Woodward N, Adler M W. Needle exchange in central London (abstract). Presented at the IVth International Conference on AIDS, Stockholm 1988; **Book 2**: 8512.

8. Ross M W. Psychological determinants of increased condom use and safer sex in homosexual men: a longitudinal study. Int J STDs and AIDS 1990; **1**: 98-101.

9. Holland J, Ramazanglu C, Scott S, Thomson R. "Don't die of ignorance - I nearly died of embarrassment": Women at risk AIDS project: condoms in context. London: Tufnell Press, 1990.

10. Chapman S, Stoker L, Ward M, Porritt D, Fahey P. Discriminant attitudes and beliefs about condoms in young, multi-partner heterosexuals. Int J STDs and AIDS 1990; **1**: 422-28.

11. Breakwell G, Fife-Shaw C R. Heterosexual anal intercourse and the risks of AIDS and HIV for 16-20 year olds. Health Educ J 1991; **5(4)**: 166-69.

12. Griffiths M. Contraceptive practices and contraceptive failures among women requesting termination or pregnancy. Br J Family Planning 1990; **16**: 16-18.

17

Family Planning and Reproductive Health Issues

Background paper and report by Marie Goldsmith, Health Education Authority, London

Other working group members were:

Nicholas Dodd (Chairperson)	*WHO*
Sanderijn van der Doef	*The Netherlands*
Tony Klouda	*UK*
Sallie Robins	*UK*
Connie Smith	*UK*
Marie-Pascale Staedel	*France*
Jorge Torgal Garcia	*Portugal*
Beate Wimmer-Puchinger	*Austria*

Introduction

Sexual health is a nebulous term. In the UK, family planners see sexual health as a component of family planning rather than treating it as an umbrella term, whereas HIV educators tend to view sexual health as a secondary and sometimes marginal consideration in HIV prevention. STDs are sometimes referred to as if they do not include HIV infection. There is thus a long way to go before the various disciplines involved in sexual health share a common understanding of sexual health promotion.

Sexual health has been defined in various ways but in most interpretations one can recognise three essential components:

- absence and avoidance of STDs and disorders which affect reproduction;
- control of fertility and avoidance of unwanted pregnancy;
- sexual expression and enjoyment without exploitation, oppression or abuse.

It is often the last of these which is neglected in health education programmes, yet this is clearly the basis for achieving the other two components of sexual health. Many now realise that a climate which celebrates, rather than restrains, sexuality in its various forms, and which acknowledges the gender power structure of heterosexual relationships, is needed to underpin efforts to achieve safer sex behaviour for prevention of disease and unintended pregnancy.

In promoting sexual health, the services for family planning, maternal and child health, and the control of STDs all have a role to play. As STDs have a major impact upon fertility and pregnancy outcome it is vital that the fertility control services and the reproductive health services play an active part in STD prevention programmes and vice versa.

There is much to be gained by adopting a holistic approach to sexual health promotion through each of these services, certainly at local level, whilst recognising that they each have their own speciality and primary focus. To date there is little evidence of this coordinated approach taking place, although secondary prevention services are integrated to differing degrees across Europe[1].

Reproductive Health Issues

It is well known that STDs often manifest themselves primarily as complications of the female reproductive tract. Emerging data suggests that even minor reproductive tract infections such as trichomoniasis may augment the transmission of HIV, which underscores the urgency of a more comprehensive approach to these infections[2].

There is also an urgent need to review the effect of spermicides on reproductive tract infections and to develop an effective virucidal method which does not cause irritation to the vaginal and rectal mucosa. Further research is needed to identify a safe and effective method within the control of women for preventing STDs and particularly HIV infection[3].

Family Planning

The public health rationale for family planning is recognised in most European countries, although contraceptive usage, unwanted pregnancy and abortion rates vary considerably, and approaches to service provision also differ.

Family planning services

In Germany gynaecologists, who are not hospital-based, are the main source of family planning advice and provision. In Italy, Spain and Sweden, midwives play a prominent role and in Britain and The Netherlands a choice exists between the family doctor, where most provision occurs (70% in UK), and a system of family planning clinics. The clinics play a valuable role for sexual health promotion as they are more popular among the young and those who are uncomfortable with the service of their family doctor, or for those who want more information and a wider choice of family planning methods. In the United States the clinic system is mainly used by those on low income and is consequently seen as a less attractive service than private doctors.

Research from the Alan Guttmacher Institute[4] showed that where young people have access to sex education and services for family planning, the rates of teenage pregnancy are lower. Similarly, Dutch research, presented by J Rademakers at the Brook Advisory Centres 1990 annual general meeting[5], showed that young family planning clinic attenders were more competent in their negotiating skills with sexual partners than girls attending abortion clinics. This illustrates the value of family planning services in enabling young people to avoid unwanted pregnancy. Similar personal skills are required when considering STD prevention in a sexual relationship.

Contraceptive usage

This varies considerably amongst countries. The International Health Foundation studied contraceptive behaviour in eight countries in Western Europe and found that where use was highest (Sweden, Denmark and Great Britain — The Netherlands was not included in the survey) reliable reversible contraceptive methods are supervised by GPs or are provided within the framework of a well-developed system of family planning clinics. These three countries also offer the least expensive range of contraceptive methods, with primary health care staff comprising the key personnel involved in contraception and family planning.

Condoms and other barrier methods were widely used in all countries except the (pre-unification) Federal Republic of Germany and France:

	Italy	France	GB	Spain	FRG	Austria	Sweden	Denmark
% using barrier methods 95% condoms	23	9	17	23	7	16	27	25

Britain is the only country of the eight surveyed where all methods are free of charge, and condoms are less expensive to buy in Britain, although several countries offer free condoms as part of AIDS education campaigns.

Many other factors affect contraceptive usage, as for example in Romania where a major problem is that actual provision of contraceptives requires hard currency. In Bulgaria it is estimated that only 5% of the population use condoms, which may be due in part to the resistance to any sexual publicity and social interventions for health education.

Abortion and unwanted pregnancy

Rates vary across Europe with Britain and Holland having the lowest teenage pregnancy rates of 14 per thousand girls aged 15-19 in The Netherlands and 45 per thousand in England and Wales (1980-81 figures)[4]. This compares with 96 per thousand in the United States, but in Romania Dr Nanu Dimitrie has estimated that one in five conceptions have been aborted, criminally, with an associated high rate of maternal mortality[6]. Even in Britain, abortion rates continue to rise, with consequent political and public concern. In 1988 there were over 120,700 teenage pregnancies in England and Wales, approximately a third of which were terminated[7].

Those presenting for abortion are prime targets for sexual health promotion, with contraception and diagnosis and treatment of STDs also being available through these services, or by easy referral to linked services.

Maternal and Child Health Services

As with the family planning services, maternal and child health services see mainly fertile women. They are therefore well placed to provide information on maternal-foetal transmission of HIV and raise awareness about early treatment of STDs to avoid reinfection and the longer term effects on fertility.

As heterosexual transmission of HIV increases in Europe, vertical transmission will become more significant in future years. Unlinked anonymous screening of pregnant women can be used to determine the prevalence of HIV in a population and thus to assess its impact on the health of both mothers and their children.

Ideally most women should have received some form of sexual health education before reaching the maternal and child health clinics, but for some these clinics may be the sole point of contact with health services. They can provide an ideal opportunity for screening for STDs, cervical smear testing, provision of contraception and sexual health promotion. Measures are essential to prevent disease transmission and progression while maintaining confidentiality, but there are several arguments both for and against routine testing for HIV infection in these settings, which are not based simply upon the seroprevalence rate in the population.

Whereas some preventable congenital infections (eg syphilis and herpes) can be treated, HIV infection for the most part cannot. The effects of knowing a positive result are not always beneficial for a pregnant woman, and the risk of her baby becoming infected may be as low as 13% in some cases[8].

Apart from unlinked anonymous screening for epidemiological reasons, only voluntary testing for HIV infection should be applied through maternal and child health services. Women should be enabled to make their own informed choices about testing, and whether or not to continue the pregnancy in the event of a positive result, whether to breast-feed, and about subsequent contraception.

However, reports suggest that prevalence rates of HIV within refusers of voluntary testing can be higher than in those who agree to be tested[1], and that women with higher risk behaviours may deny this risk and not agree to testing[9].

STD Services

Britain is fortunate in having a long-established system of freely accessible clinics for the diagnosis, treatment and contact tracing of STDs, through the genitourinary medicine (GUM) departments of local hospitals. In some other European countries, the dermato-venereology departments of major hospitals bear this responsibility and in others GPs play a key role in STD control. Contact tracing is carried out routinely for some STDs apart from HIV but much of the experience of STD personnel in contact tracing could be transferred to HIV prevention and education[1].

WHO Recommendations

The World Health Organisation has recommended incorporation of HIV/STD prevention into family planning (FP) and maternal and child health (MCH) programmes as a fundamental step in pursuing the goals of HIV and STD prevention and control[10]. Their recommendations include:

- Strengthening the infrastructure of MCH/FP programmes.
- Strengthening the training of MCH/FP service providers.
- Improving knowledge and attitudes to HIV among MCH/FP workers.
- Strengthening the counselling and communication skills of MCH/FP workers.
- Strengthening MCH/FP information, education and communication programmes to include an AIDS component.

The Benefits of Coordinated Sexual Health Promotion Services

Where family planning and reproductive health services are established, they provide an infrastructure for STD/HIV health education and broaden the outlets beyond the principal services of GUM and dermato-venereology. Similarly an infrastructure of STD centres could provide additional access points for contraceptive and reproductive health education. Most consumers would welcome the convenience of being able to address their sexual health needs under one roof, and this can result in cost savings for the health service.

A Birth Control Trust survey[11] at two London clinics found evidence for this: 10.4% of women (29.6% of those under 20 years of age) visiting the GUM clinic were at risk of unwanted pregnancy, and 1.8% of women visiting the family planning clinic had symptoms of genitourinary infection. The researchers recommended that GUM clinics take contraceptive histories and offer some contraceptive services, and that family planning clinics provide at least diagnosis and referral for STDs. In fact, some respondents at both clinics had expected to receive counselling in all aspects of sexual health. In both clinics, a third of women had not seen their GP within the last year, and 25% at the GUM clinic and 21% at the family planning clinic were visiting a clinic for the first time.

However, lines of responsibility and accountability can become confused where local programmes and services are integrated but programmes and policies are separated at a central or higher level. Integration of two or more disciplines can also lead to dilution of expertise, loss of specialisation and lower standards of service. Coordination, rather than integration, may therefore be the best option.

Consultations in family planning and reproductive health services

In sexual health promotion, interventions involving small groups or one-to-one situations are most effective in achieving behaviour change. Mass media campaigns can achieve significant awareness levels but these need to link with face-to-face opportunities for education, as for example during the consultations through the family planning and reproductive health services.

Health workers in family planning and maternity services constitute a large pool of expertise in dealing with sensitive health issues around sexuality, contraception, and reproductive health. Health promotion about HIV and other STDs is a natural extension of their role, as similar skills are required for giving advice on disease prevention and for developing a sexual counselling role. Once trained in STD/HIV health promotion skills, the workers in these services may be able to provide awareness training for other health and social workers or community groups on a cascade model.

The regular check-ups which some women have for their contraceptive method offer an opportunity to build up a rapport with the family planning worker. A similar situation might apply with regular antenatal and child health checks. This rapport allows the worker to gain personal knowledge of the client, which is useful when needing to ask delicate or intimate questions. Discussions about contraception and pregnancy can lead naturally into more sensitive areas of sexual relationships and their impact on health.

When sexual behaviour is discussed in consultations with these services, it would seem unrealistic and even negligent to talk only in terms of pregnancy and fertility control without reference to STDs, their implications for fertility, and how to protect against them.

These services could provide pre-test counselling for the worried well to relieve the demand on HIV/STD treatment services. Some STDs could be diagnosed and possibly treated through the family planning and reproductive health services, although it is essential to perform sexual health checks to detect other infections which may be masked or asymptomatic. Contact tracing may present difficulties, although contacts may prefer to be seen at these centres rather than in GUM/venereology departments. Testing for HIV infection presents particular problems (see above, page 123).

A word of caution is warranted, however — family planning and reproductive health is seen by some as the positive side to sexual health, whereas HIV/STD prevention may be associated with some more negative aspects. This could result in even more stigma being associated with STDs. If STD and HIV counselling is found to be on offer at family planning or reproductive health centres, there mayb be hostile reactions from the public, and some may be discouraged from attending[12]. Extra sensitivity is needed in addressing STDs with family planning and reproductive health clients who are not expecting consultation on this subject, unlike attenders at STD clinics.

Condom promotion

Family planning services provide an established outlet for condom distribution in some countries, and in Britain the family planning clinics and GUM clinics are the only source of free condoms, apart from a few specific projects working with particular target groups for HIV prevention.

Family planning workers are familiar with condoms and experienced at instruction in their use. As condoms can be 98% effective (for contraception) when used carefully and consistently, family planning workers can do much to promote their dual function for preventing pregnancy, HIV and other STDs. However, some family planning workers may not readily advise condom use because it has been considered a less effective contraceptive than the oral contraceptive and other methods. Conflicting interests may arise when the most effective contraceptive method is required at the same time as protection against HIV.

Advising condom use for prophylaxis and a more effective method for contraception raises dilemmas, not only in persuading clients to practise such "belt and braces" tactics, but also in terms of cost. There may be difficulties in providing condoms free to the consumer for both prophylaxis and contraception. In the UK, GPs cannot prescribe condoms free to the consumer, but can do this for medical methods of contraception.

The Working Group's Recommendations

Discussions during the workshop centred around ways of utilising and improving family planning and reproductive health provision to encompass broader sexual health promotion within services. The following recommendations form an edited version of the report produced during the workshop itself, but with little change to the content.

Skilled, appropriate family planning can help individuals make a personal risk-benefit analysis, choose from the available contraceptive methods, and become motivated for their continuing careful use. However it is clear that some individuals do not live in social environments which support the use of contraception. It is also clear that such environments may not support independent decision-making about sexual interaction that is safe from unwanted pregnancy, STDs, HIV or the abuse of power. Contraceptive providers should therefore develop programmes within the framework of sexual health which address these issues in the communities they serve. This requires the establishment and further development of client-centred services. Provider-led agendas cannot meet the needs of those most vulnerable and least able to contact services.

A variety of sources of contraception are needed, even in countries with well-established medical primary care services, to provide for those (especially adolescents) who will not consult their "family doctor" on issues of sexuality.

The inclusion of a broader agenda of sexual health promotion within the work of contraceptive providers should not need a giant step. Women and men attending for contraceptive services have, to some extent, acknowledged that they are sexually active or planning to become so, and are seeking professional services. However, some issues of policy and practice will have to be addressed, within family planning and reproductive health services and at national policy-making levels, for progress to be made in fully using the existing services to promote sexual health.

Building healthy public policy

All countries should have a comprehensive public health policy on sexual health.

Part of this overall policy would clearly define a broader range of health promotion, health education and service activities in regard to sexual health. This could be carried out by family planning and reproductive health services as they are currently constituted, or if needed, within a restructured programme.

Such a policy would have to take into account a number of key points including:

- Confidentiality, respect for individuals and free and informed choices.

- Free and easy access to a number of alternative services acceptable to different population groups.

- Assurance of the required funding, and the necessary national and local structures to support the implementation of a national public health policy on sexual health.

- The vital role of sex education in schools in developing communication skills, personal sexual responsibility, positive attitudes towards sexuality, and a greater willingness to seek professional assistance.

- Wider and more targetted advertising of where services are available.

- Integration rather than fragmentation of services so that ideally all sexual health issues can be dealt with under one roof — whether "family planning" or "reproductive health".

- The research needed to underpin promotion of sexual health, for example on the interactions between contraceptive methods and HIV transmission.

- The need to maintain high standards of practice and skills for the full range of counselling and contraceptive services.

Two initial steps are vital in order to stimulate the development of a public health policy on sexual health:

- Firstly, politicians and other decision makers must be convinced that proactive promotion of sexual health and prevention of STDs, unwanted pregnancy and psychosexual problems and their social repercussions are more cost-effective for the tax-payer (consumer) than attempting to cure or alleviate these problems after their occurrence. (These "secondary" services will still be required, but in the long term to a lesser degree.) Research demonstrating this for family planning services[13] could be replicated for sexual health. One way may be to set up and evaluate model sexual health promotion services.

- Secondly, the existing family planning and reproductive health teams should be fully involved in managing the change to achieve the fullest definition and provision of sexual health promotion. In this way both benefits to clients and rewards to providers can be maximised.

Creating supportive environments and strengthening community action

In broadening the scope of family planning and reproductive health services to include a full range of sexual health promotion, education and service activities, a number of aspects relating to the creation of supportive social, community and service environments need to be considered. These include acknowledgement of the following:

- The special needs for women to receive sexual health promotion services in a safe environment that is respectful of their needs.

- The importance of developing further and using non-medical models in addition to medical models of practice.

126

- The need for services to seek and obtain the expertise of a variety of health and non-health professionals and peer group workers in addressing the social and community environments.

- The requirement for sexual health promotion activities to be sensitive to client preferences as regards the sex of the provider and to the needs of different ethnic and cultural groups.

- The need for consumer-oriented services, ie services aware of and responsive to the diverse communities they serve. This can only be realised through greater involvement of consumers in the design of services and greater consultation with the community on decisions about service provision.

- The need to foster non-exploitative community action, harnessing peer group sexual health promotion and education.

- The importance of services engendering positive attitudes towards sexuality.

- The requirement for non-threatening and non-judgemental attitudes on the part of service providers.

- The service providers' own need for a supportive environment to enable them to attain high levels of achievement and commitment.

- The need to raise awareness among professional peers of both the importance and the location of sexual health promotion services.

Developing personal skills

Training underpins the ability of family planning and reproductive health workers to communicate effectively with clients in matters relating to sexual health. To be effective, training will require the assistance of appropriate trainers with expertise in participatory and experiential learning methods and techniques necessary for mastering communication skills.

Training should be for all staff, should be relevant to their roles, and should emphasise their contribution to the work of the team. The goals of such training should be:

- To help workers to become more aware of and comfortable with their own sexuality and that of others so that they are enabled to provide help in a non-judgemental manner.

- To increase knowledge on STDs, including HIV, and their prevention; to explore, and challenge where necessary, attitudes to people with HIV, AIDS or STDs and drug users; to enable risk assessment for unplanned pregnancy, HIV and STD infection.

- To improve counselling techniques and enhance communication and negotiating skills of themselves and of their clients.

Re-orienting services

For sexual health promotion to be effective, all activities must be more sensitive to the variety of cultural needs and expectations of clients. Client-oriented services should have the following characteristics:

- An agreed framework for sexual health promotion activities.

- A management system which encourages teamwork and an inter-disciplinary approach to service provision.

- A clear set of objectives and activities based on community needs, which will be continuously monitored, evaluated and re-assessed.

- The resources required to carry out planned activities.

- Managerial training aimed at service re-orientation, and assistance in identifying the sources of such training, eg production of a directory.

- The removal of barriers to the use of services, especially by "hard to reach" consumers, for example by setting opening and closing times convenient for clients and staff.

- Easy access for those with disabilities and consideration of the needs of men and black and minority ethnic people.

- An assurance of the quality of the associated secondary referral services.

- A definition of the limits or boundaries of work within the services, according to the availability of resources.

References

1. WHO Regional Office for Europe. Review of areas of integration between STD services and AIDS prevention and control programmes. EUR/ICP/GPA 079 A. Copenhagen: WHO, 1990.

2. Manoka A T, et al. Non-ulcerative sexually transmitted diseases as risk factors for HIV infection (abstract). Fifth International Conference on AIDS in Africa, Zaire, 1990.

3. Elias C. Sexually transmitted diseases and the reproductive health of women in developing countries. Working Paper No. 5. New York: Population Council, 1991.

4. Jones E F, Forrest J D, Henshaw S K, Silverman J, Torres A. Pregnancy, contraception and family planning services in industrialised countries. New Haven/London: Yale University Press, 1989.

5. Godlee F. Dutch example on teenage sexuality (news). Br Med J 1990; **301**: 511.

6. Bromham D R. What will we do in 1992? (Editorial). Br J Family Plan 1990; **16**: 81-83.

7. Estaugh V, Wheatley J. Family planning and family well-being. Occasional paper 12. London: Family Policy Studies Centre, 1990.

8. European Collaborative Study. Children born to women with HIV-1 infection: natural history and risk of transmission. Lancet 1991; **337**: 253-260.

9. Berrier J, Sperling R, Preisinger J, Evans V, Mason J, Walther V. HIV/AIDS education in a prenatal clinic: an assessment. AIDS Education and Prevention 1991; **3(2)**: 100-117.

10. World Health Organisation. AIDS prevention: guidelines for MCH/FP programme managers. Geneva: WHO 1990.

11. Queen H F, Ward H, Smith C, Woodroffe C. Women's health: potential for better coordination of services. Genitourin Med 1991; **67**: 215-219.

12. Barbour R S, MacIntyre S, McIlwaine G, Wilson E. Uptake of AIDS counselling and testing at a Scottish family planning clinic. Brit J Fam Plann 1989; **15**: 61-62.

13. Laing W A. Family planning: the benefits and costs. London: Policy Studies Institute, 1982.

18

Minority Ethnic People

Background paper and report by Rinske van Duifhuizen, Co-ordinator, AIDS prevention for migrants, Dutch National Committee on AIDS Control

Other working group members were:

James Hospedales (Chairperson)	*Trinidad*
J Wagdi Al-Jeddahwi	*Sweden*
Mehboob Dada	*UK*
Huseyin Demirkan	*Switzerland*
Simon Hall	*UK*
Mary Haour-Knipe	*Switzerland*
Jayshree Pillaye	*UK*
Anne Solberg	*Norway*
Márta Váczi	*Hungary*
Sali-Ann Walker	*UK*

1.   Introduction

This section provides theoretical and background information about minority ethnic people as an introduction to considering the practicalities of HIV/STD prevention* for this specific target group.

1.1   What is meant by minority ethnic people?

Minority ethnic groups are usually taken to mean groups of people who migrated to a country, originally for economic reasons, and at the time of immigration had a low socio-economic position within the receiving country. This position meant that these groups could not fully participate in society and were often disadvantaged.

The working group used a broad definition of minority ethnic people: *minority ethnic people are people with a significantly different cultural and linguistic background, compared to the majority of the population.* This concept of "minority ethnic people" includes asylum seekers, refugees, (im)migrants, migrant-workers, gypsies and people with no legal right to stay in the receiving country as well as Black and other minority groups born within the country but descended from an immigrant group.

Clearly, therefore "minority ethnic people" do not exist as a homogeneous group. There are many differences between and within minority ethnic groups. None the less, the concept is useful when considering the appropriate targeting of HIV/STD prevention.

1.2   Demographic situation in Europe

The percentage of "foreigners" within the total population in Europe differs from country to country and is available in official statistics, though it must be recognised that many minority ethnic people may be nationals

---

* The chapter is confined largely to HIV prevention, for purely pragmatic reasons because experience with targeted prevention directed towards ethnic minority people started in most cases with HIV.

of the country concerned while, conversely, "foreigners" may have a similar cultural and linguistic background to the host population. In the UK it is 4.7%, in The Netherlands 5.1%, in West Germany 7.6%, in Norway 4.3%, in France 8.0% and in Belgium 8.7% (Eurostat 1989). As well as the numbers, the countries of origin of the most important groups vary widely for different European countries, as shown in Table 1. Former colonial relations have played an important role in migration processes, as for example over 40% of the foreign population in France comes from North Africa.

**Table 1: The three largest EEC and non-EEC ethnic minority groups
in selected countries**

Country	EEC ethnic minorities	Non-EEC ethnic minorities
Belgium	Italy, 241,000 France, 91,400 The Netherlands, 60,5000	Morocco, 135,000 Turkey, 79,500 United States, 11,600
France[a]	Portugal, 751,300 Italy, 277,100 Spain, 267,000	Algeria, 820,900 Morocco, 516,400 Tunisia, 202,600
Germany	Italy, 508,700 Greece, 274,800 Austria, 155,100	Turkey, 1,523,700 Yugoslavia, 579,100 Morocco, 52,100
The Netherlands	Germany, 40,300 United Kingdom, 37,400 Belgium, 23,100	Turkey, 176,500 Morocco, 139,200 Yugoslavia, 12,100
Norway	Denmark, 18,100 United Kingdom, 13,200 Germany, 4,300	Pakistan, 11,100 United States, 10,100 Vietnam, 6,500
Sweden	Denmark, 25,600 Germany, 11,900 United Kingdom, 9,300	Finland, 127,900 Yugoslavia, 38,900 Norway, 28,600
Switzerland	Italy, 382,300 Spain, 114,00 Germany, 80,300	Yugoslavia, 100,700 Turkey, 56,800 United States, 9,300

a) 1985 data   Source: SOPEMI 1989

Most of the minority ethnic groups in Europe have a very young age structure. The vast majority are under forty years old, eg. 95% in France, 70% in Spain and 90% (under 44) in Italy (SOPEMI 1989). This is due to the fact that original migrants are for the most part workers in their prime, often single men.

1.3   *General trends of international migration*

The main feature of international migration in recent years has been the growth of migratory flows especially of asylum seekers and refugees (see Table 2), together with the arrival of people from Central and Eastern European countries and ongoing family reunification.

A second important feature is the changing patterns of emigration and return migration. For years, migration within Europe took place from South to North but this is changing with the economic development of the Southern European countries. Emigration from the traditional sending countries continues but at a reduced rate. In contrast, movement of skilled workers between the highly industrialised countries is increasing (SOPEMI 1989).

Further points of note include that, despite all efforts to control incoming people, illegal immigration persists. Foreign populations are growing within European countries, posing challenges for the social and economic integration of migrants. Policies aimed at influencing migratory flows are very difficult to implement in view of the complexity of the problem, taking in demographic, historical, cultural and financial factors, and the different stages of the migratory process in different European countries.

Table 2: Asylum seekers in selected European OECD countries

Countries	1983	1988	1989[a]	Mean annual increase 1983-1988, %
Austria	5868	15790	18300	21.9
Belgium	2937	5078	8115	11.6
Denmark	800	4700	4600	42.5
France	22285	34253	61200	9.0
Germany	19737	103076	121318	39.2
Greece	450	6950[b]		98.2[c]
Italy	3050	11050[b]		38.0[c]
The Netherlands	2000	7500	14000	30.3
Norway	150	6602	4400	113.2
Portugal	1500	450[b]		-26.0[c]
Spain	1400	2500[b]		15.6[c]
Sweden	4000	19600	32000	37.4
Switzerland	7886	16726	24500	16.2
United Kingdom	3550	5100		7.5

a) *provisional data*
b) *1987 data*
c) *1983-87*

Source: National statistics

Recent political events, particularly in Central and Eastern Europe, must be taken into account as they will lead to new migration movements in the future. Continued opening of the frontiers of Central and Eastern European Countries and liberalisation of their economies is likely and will have its consequences.

The freedom of movement for workers within the European Communities from 1993 will probably cause increased mobility amongst workers at all levels of skill.

2. Why are Minority Ethnic People Important for AIDS Prevention?

This section analyses the most important specific characteristics of this target group which must be taken into account when one is dealing with HIV/STD prevention.

2.1 Demographic and socio-economic characteristics

The relatively young age structure of most minority ethnic groups, as mentioned above, is an important factor to bear in mind since AIDS and STDs particularly concern young people (20-40). Additionally, higher birth rates amongst minority ethnic groups have the effect of maintaining the youthfulness of this group in comparison to the general population.

Another important characteristic of minority ethnic groups is high unemployment rates, although this varies very widely between groups and countries. In most European countries minority ethnic people belong to the low socio-economic classes: poorly educated, with bad housing conditions, high unemployment, over-represented among low paid workers, and with disproportionately high unemployment among women and young people.

For some European countries, unemployment among the foreign population is still increasing, or is decreasing less than for the national population. The circumstances of different nationality groups can contrast markedly, as for example in Belgium where Italians make up 38% of foreign unemployment but only 22% of the total foreign labour force.

Most of the minority ethnic groups are concentrated in the biggest cities Europe, where housing shortages are generally marked. The financially weakest groups, in which ethnic minorities are over-represented, mostly have to wait long periods for housing and often end up living in low quality and sub-standard housing.

2.2   *Epidemiological trends*

Although this chapter focuses on the European situation, reference will also be made to the situation in the United States since there is extensive published data about HIV prevalence in US minority ethnic populations, particularly for Black people and Hispanic people (the two largest minority ethnic groups in that country). It should, however, be noted that the situation in the United States is not readily comparable to that in Europe. Important differences include: totally different ethnic groups; differing socio-economic situations; and wide-scale IV drug use within ethnic groups in the US which does not reflect patterns of drug use in Europe. But it is equally true for both regions that health problems are harder to address among the lower socio-economic classes than others and that minority ethnic people are over-represented in these sections of society. It is therefore important to be aware of the US experience and to try to prevent its happening again in Europe.

Black people and Hispanic people represent only 12.0% and 6.0% respectively of the US population, but some 26% and 13% of all people with AIDS. The age distribution and exposure categories of cases show significant differences by race/ethnicity, as shown in Table 3[1]. While 76% of White adult/adolescent AIDS cases are attributed to homosexually acquired HIV infection, the corresponding figures for Black and Hispanic people are only 36% and 40%. Intravenous drug use accounted for about 40% of cases among the latter groups.

Similarly, for paediatric AIDS cases (younger than 13 years) a higher proportion of cases among Black and Hispanic people than among Whites are attributable to maternal risk status or infection. In particular, data not shown in the table shows a high proportion of mothers using drugs or having had sex with drug users among these cases.

While less than 5% of adult/adolescent White AIDS patients are women, the figure is 18% for Blacks and 12% for Hispanics.

No comparable study on HIV or AIDS prevalence by ethnicity in different countries has been undertaken in Europe. Although the nationality of people with AIDS has been registered in most European countries, these data are mostly not published because of fear of stigmatisation of certain groups.

In the UK, known Black, Asian and Oriental people comprised 7% of the total number of reported people with AIDS, with ethnicity unknown for 9% of cases[2]. Two thirds of people presumed to have contracted HIV abroad are black heterosexuals (Dada, personal communication).

In Belgium almost 50% (354) of the diagnosed people with AIDS were foreign, and of these only 24% lived in Belgium. More than 75% of these foreign people with AIDS came from Africa and in 70% of the cases the transmission mode was heterosexual contact[3].

In The Netherlands 20% of reported people with AIDS are foreign nationals (272). Of these people 45% (125) came from other European countries, 15% from Latin-America (40), 13% from the United States (35), 10% from Africa and 10% from Asia (National Committee on AIDS Control, October 1990).

During the workshop there was considerable discussion of *the need for epidemiological data as a basis for drawing up specific HIV prevention strategies for minority ethnic people.* Hitherto, statistics on the ethnic origin of people with HIV/AIDS have been scarce, or not published if available. However, in some countries these figures are necessary to convince policy makers of the importance of specific AIDS prevention work for minority ethnic groups. *These data must be collected with great care and used responsibly. Lack of data should not be used as an excuse for not doing prevention work in this area.*

**Table 3: AIDS cases by exposure category and race/ethnicity,
reported up to November 1990, USA**

	White, not hispanic	Black, not hispanic	Hispanic	Total[a]
Adult/adolescent cases (numbers)	85884	43094	24269	154791
Exposure categories (%):-				
Male homo/bisexual	76	36	40	59
IVDU	8	39	40	22
Haemophilia	7	7	6	7
Heterosexual contact (US)[b]	2	7	6	4
Heterosexual contact (Pattern II country)[c]	*	5	*	1
Blood or tissue recipient	3	1	2	2
Other/undetermined	2	5	5	4
Paediatric cases (numbers)	586	1412	710	2734
Exposure categories (%):-				
Mother with/at risk for HIV infection	60	92	85	83
Other/undetermined	40	8	14	16

* *less than 0.1%*   Source: Ref 1.

a) *Includes other/unknown racial/ethnic groups.*
b) *Heterosexual contact with person in recognised exposure category or known to be HIV positive, risk unspecified.*
c) *Born in Pattern II country or heterosexual contact with person born in Pattern II country.*

2.3 Travel restrictions

"The key to block HIV at borders is mandatory testing for seropositivity, which creates a number of problems and is subject to numerous abuses. Uniform HIV testing is not required by any of the European countries, but in practice it may be "offered" to certain people, most often asylum seekers and refugees, without the recipient knowing that he or she has the right to refuse. Some require obligatory testing for certain categories (eg. students). One major result of this sort of policy is to create a black market in negative test certificates".[4]

The working group was concerned that some countries try to tackle the problem of AIDS by trying to block it at the border. Travel restrictions are likely to be issued because the ancestral link of minority ethnic people to their countries of origin and their links with travel and migration.

The working group agreed with the conclusions of Gilmore[5] that *travel restrictions are a not justifiable measure to prevent HIV transmission.* They are impractical, ineffective, wasteful, discriminatory, costly and harmful.

2.4 Minority ethnic people as a specific target group

The general, basic premise of health promotion is that *it is the responsibility of every country to ensure that all segments of the population receive the information necessary to prevent HIV transmission in an appropriate way.* In this respect, the duties imposed upon states by international human rights instruments do not distinguish between nationals and non-nationals. Indeed, the exclusion of one population group from access to health information is considered as a form of unfair discrimination.

Moreover, the US experience shows that minority ethnic communities are relatively harder hit by AIDS than the majority community. Although the situation is unclear, the same may be true in Europe or may become so in the near future. There are indications that some minority ethnic groups in Europe are already relatively more affected than the majority population, for example Cape Verdians in The Netherlands and people from Zaire in Belgium. Such groups tend to come from high HIV prevalence areas. However, on evidence so far available, most minority ethnic people in Europe should generally not be seen as a *risk group* but as *groups with specific prevention needs* deriving from cultural and language differences.

Sexual health promotion must take into account that migration and travel are of importance for the spread of AIDS and other STDs, and that this relation is undeniable[5,6]. People travel abroad and have sexual contacts and use drugs while abroad. But this should *not* lead to stigmatisation of travellers or more specifically of migrants and refugees.

3.   Health Promotion Experiences

3.1   Experiences to date

Integral AIDS prevention activities were launched the early eighties in a number of European countries, but the first national AIDS prevention programmes directed towards minority ethnic people were established in 1988.

Most of the primary efforts to reach minority ethnic people in European countries consisted of translating different materials (leaflets, brochures, posters) into community languages. Now, more and more countries have become aware that this is not always an appropriate method, for example where literacy is not the primary focus and/or oral traditions predominate. More intensive activities in which minority ethnic people are involved and participate actively have been started.

To give an impression of what is going on examples will be given for Belgium, Hungary, Norway, Sweden, Switzerland, The Netherlands and the United Kingdom.

Belgium: In the city of Brussels a local non-governmental organisation (Service Social des Etrangers) is coordinating AIDS prevention activities for minority ethnic people. The activities are integrated in more general information programmes for these groups. Organisations working for minority ethnic people are provided with materials and advice on how to organise educational meetings. The service has produced materials in different languages and a multi-cultural series of slides. Different organisations are involved in preparing and implementing the prevention activities, and there is close collaboration with minority ethnic "group leaders"[3].

Norway: Of a population of 4 million inhabitants about 200,000 persons have a non-Norwegian background. In addition to the HIV-STD prevention measures undertaken by the primary health services in the different Norwegian municipalities, since 1989/90 the Directorate of Health has supported pilot projects aiming at specific information activities in cooperation with immigrant organisations, as well as resource persons both within and outside organised foreign language settings. The idea behind these projects is to draw on the cultural and linguistic competence of the various minority ethnic groups in preparing and planning informational activities.

Strategies for the work include development of networks, peer-education, and outreach activities as well as developing of materials (Solberg, personal communication).

The Netherlands: In The Netherlands there has been a structured national programme since 1989 for AIDS prevention activities directed towards migrants, co-ordinated by the National Committee on AIDS Control. The programme focusses on development of materials, development of educational methods and network development. There is a national working group in which organisations of and for migrants are represented.

A basic point of departure for every project is the active participation of minority ethnic people during all phases of the project — preparation, implementation and evaluation.

Specific items and media for minority ethnic people are integrated in the national mass campaigns for the general public. In addition there are specific projects directed towards different ethnic groups eg. training of ethnic group educators, ethnic minority hotlines and the development of audiotapes and videotapes[7].

Sweden: Of a total population of 8.4 million, Sweden counts a minority ethnic population (immigrants and refugees) of 1 million people.

Different materials (brochures, overheads, slides, videotapes, posters, advertisements and exhibitions) are produced in eleven languages: English, French, German, Spanish, Arabic, Finnish, Yugoslavian, Greek, Polish, Persian and Swedish. Specific activities such as mass campaigns and a AIDS information centre are undertaken (Al-Jeddahwi, personal communication).

Switzerland: In January 1991, a specific prevention project for the Turkish, Spanish and Portuguese population started within the Federal Office of Public Health in Berne, in collaboration with the Swiss Aids Foundation. This pilot project should be extended to other large foreign populations. It is conducted by members of the concerned minority ethnic communities in order to reach as many people as possible within these groups, by providing specific items and materials, and encouraging social events related to AIDS prevention in Switzerland. The target groups participate when developing materials and methodologies (Demirkan, personal communication).

United Kingdom: In the United Kingdom the Health Education Authority (HEA) plays a key role in developing strategies to reach black and minority ethnic communities.

The HEA works closely together with local, regional and national organisations (including the voluntary sector). The United Kingdom started in 1987 with an extension of the existing National AIDS Helpline, with a series of taped messages in various community languages and in 1988 a series of AIDS information leaflets. Later, special advisers were employed at the helpline to provide HIV/AIDS information and personalised counselling in a variety of languages, largely Asian ones.

The Department of Health provides financial support for nationally based voluntary groups such as the Black HIV and AIDS Network. The HEA's programme for the future will focus on increased mass media campaigns, local and community work and inter-personal approaches that are specific and relevant to the needs of black and minority ethnic communities in England (Dada, personal communication).

As well as these examples, the working group knew of prevention activities for minority ethnic people in *Germany, France* and *Italy* which were becoming more and more concretely structured.

3.2   Problems encountered

The problems faced by people working on AIDS prevention for minority ethnic groups can be grouped round several themes.

Research: Everybody working in this specific field finds a lack of relevant data. Basic research on knowledge, attitudes and sexual behaviour is not available. Knowledge on media use of minority ethnic groups and evaluation studies of different prevention methods (process and effectiveness) are also lacking. The need for more qualitative and quantitative research is evident.

The prevention message: By this the working group did not mean only the content of the message, which must clearly be the same as for anyone else. But the way of communicating the message must be culturally adapted. How can the message be made appropriate for minority ethnic people? How can stigmatisation issues be dealt with?

Policy making: Policy makers do not always consider minority ethnic people as an important target group for AIDS prevention. Minority ethnic people are often neither represented at the level of decision making nor consulted in later stages.

Money and personnel: A consequence of the above point seems to be that there is little money and few personnel available for specific activities directed towards minority ethnic people. Although it is accepted that in the long term it is desirable to integrate activities into existing programmes, financial incentives incentives are needed to start up projects. In many countries there is also a need for a source of coordination and support for activities directed towards this specific group.

Materials and methodologies: Several problems are faced in the process of developing materials and methodologies. These include how to set priorities, define objectives, choose target groups, pre-test materials and involve minority ethnic people? Another important problem is an insufficient knowledge on the part of intermediaries of basic facts about the traditions and cultural background of different minority ethnic groups. The last point to mention here is the need for wider exchange of developed materials and methods so that not everybody has to re-invent the wheel.

3.3 International cooperation

There are of course many existing (incidental) bilateral contacts between European and non-European countries, but probably these can become more effective when placed on a more structured basis.

One of the first international bodies to select minority ethnic people as a sub-group which needed to be studied was the European Communities[4]. Among the conclusions of the first exploratory study conducted was a great need for coordination. Many people in different countries were working in isolation on comparable topics and it would be beneficial for more to be done in building alliances between them. Possibilities for exchange of materials and experiences need to be explored[4].

In October 1990 the National Committee on AIDS Control of The Netherlands started a project on "AIDS and Mobility" on behalf of the European region of WHO. Within this project migrants, refugees and asylum seekers are seen as important target groups alongside other travellers. A report on the first inventory phase of this project has been published and implementation of the main project started in June 1991.

4. Discussion

The group confined its discussion of sexual health promotion to *education concerning sexual behaviour*, and spoke mostly about AIDS prevention, because of the experiences of the participants in this field. The discussion points are grouped around several themes.

4.1 Target groups, priorities, objectives

Several criteria can be considered in identifying a target group: the size, level of knowledge, sexual behaviour, drug consumption patterns, prevalence of AIDS/STDs, media use, information needs and cultural background and level of organisation of the group. These criteria are not only in the case of minority ethnic people but must be used for every target group within a health promotion programme.

Generally speaking, the objectives of AIDS prevention are usually:

- To raise the interest of the target group in AIDS as an issue that concerns them;
- To prevent (further) HIV-transmission;
- To prevent negative social consequences, eg discrimination.

These objectives are appropriate for minority ethnic people, as for other target groups. The first objective is of especial importance because members of ethnic groups often do not identify themselves with AIDS prevention messages and see it as a problem of the majority population.

4.2 Development of materials

Most countries started AIDS prevention for minority ethnic people by translating general brochures. The working group did not consider this an appropriate way to inform minority ethnic people since the translations were often very technical and difficult to read and some terms do not even exist in other languages. In most cases minority ethnic people need more (audio)visual materials.

Stigmatisation is sometimes difficult to deal with, but can be prevented by involving members of the minority ethnic groups in the process of development of materials (during the development, pre-test, distribution and evaluation phases).

Every member of the population needs to be able to identify with health promotion messages and materials. Thus general HIV/AIDS prevention materials need to be "multicultural and anti-racist" and so that such identification is possible for ethnic minority people too.

4.3 Development of methodologies

The working group distinguished methodologies on different levels according to the targets of the strategy: mass media, group education and individual education.

Several countries have good experiences with group education through members of minority groups (peer-educators), with using the specific "ethnic" media and with AIDS hotlines for different minority ethnic groups.

When discussing how to deal with homosexuality within prevention activities for minority ethnic people, the working-group talked a lot about the (very Western) concept of homosexuality. The group concluded that most of the time it is easier to talk about different sexual techniques without using the word homosexuality. Often minority ethnic people do not consider themselves as homosexuals although they do have sexual contact with people of the same sex. In consequence these people are difficult to reach through "homo-specific" activities and channels, so within general prevention programmes attention must be drawn to this too. Experience has shown that it is often difficult for people to talk about homosexual behaviour within a group, but this is easier in individual contacts (for example following a group session or via an anonymous hotline). It also came up that research in different countries has suggested that anal intercourse occurs quite often within heterosexual relations for various reasons.

The importance of the ethnicity and gender of counsellors was discussed. There are disadvantages (eg social control) and advantages (eg ease of communication) in having a counsellor of the same ethnic background and/or gender as the client. Clients should be offered a counsellor of the same ethnic background, so that they can make a choice.

It is always most effective to combine different methodologies. This general health education principle counts equally for minority ethnic people and can increase the breadth of the target group reached.

4.4 Network development

A good working network forms the basis of successful prevention strategies and in the case of HIV prevention should include statutory and non-statutory organisations. Existing formal networks for minority ethnic people must also be used for AIDS/STD-prevention. However, these are very different in each country and cannot be described in detail here.

Institutions on different levels (local, regional, national) must be involved to reach members of minority ethnic groups with AIDS prevention. Involvement of community-based organisations is virtually a pre-condition for obtaining the commitment of the target group and implementing projects in an appropriate way. It was suggested that informal networks also play an important role for AIDS prevention but experiences in this field were not presented within the working group.

Co-operation in prevention with the countries of origin of minority ethnic groups is rare. However, there were good experiences reported from the Caribbean region of using materials produced in the country of origin of minority ethnic people. The working group concluded that co-operation with countries of origin is a worthwhile adjunct to working together with people of the target group within the receiving country as a means of obtaining information and developing culturally appropriate methods.

4.5 Research

As mentioned in paragraph 3.2 there is a great need for research since existing research data on minority ethnic groups are scarce. Minority ethnic people are often not involved in general research on sexual behaviour related to AIDS and other STDs. There is some useful information derived from experience and process evaluations, but this usually cannot be generalised for a given population.

4.6 International co-operation

Despite existing EC and WHO projects on minority ethnic people, improved international co-operation is still needed. AIDS prevention for migrants is a field in which intra-European co-operation is not only indicated but essential. The need for a central reference point and data bank of information at the European level emerged repeatedly during the workshop.

4.7   Influence of travel in the future

New migration flows can be expected as a result of the forthcoming freedom of movement for workers within the EC and recent political events in central and Eastern Europe. Hitherto most central and Eastern European countries have been considered low prevalence areas compared to Western European but this may change rapidly if prevention activities are not undertaken. The first priority is to document the state of the art of health promotion in central and Eastern Europe and the patterns of trans-border crossing with Western European countries. The working group was particularly concerned at anecdotal reports of international trade in women and male and female prostitution for economic reasons.

5.   Recommendations

- Fear of stigmatisation of minority ethnic people must not lead to failure to undertake health education for this target group. It is possible to develop appropriate prevention activities without stigmatising people.
- It is a responsibility of every government to inform every inhabitant of their country about significant risks to health.
- Minority ethnic people should be consulted and involved in AIDS prevention programmes from the earliest possible stage.
- Literal translations of brochures aimed at the majority population of a country are considered as inappropriate for minority ethnic people. Materials cannot simply be transposed from one group to another. When developing materials a greater emphasis is needed on (audio)visual materials.
- Specific subgroups within minority ethnic populations must be targetted: as different audiences eg students, asylum-seekers, illegal immigrants, seasonal workers; and as people who may engage in specific risk behaviours eg men who have sex with men, drug-users, prostitutes and their clients. The needs of women have to be addressed too.
- The group reiterated that travel and immigration restrictions are not a justifiable measure to prevent AIDS/STD transmission. Mandatory testing for incoming migrants is impractical, ineffective, wasteful, discriminating, costly and harmful.

The group's key conclusions presented to the closing plenary of the workshop were that:

1. Sound policy making and planning of health promotion requires better quality information and data (particularly epidemiological data) on the health status of minority ethnic people. This data should be collected and used with proper safeguards against abuse such as measures discriminating against minority ethnic groups and foreigners.
2. Sexual health promotion activities for minority ethnic people should be accurate, appropriate, culturally and linguistically sensitive, with a greater emphasis on oral/audio/visual methodologies that are evaluated to assess appropriateness and impact and to avoid duplication of earlier mistakes.
3. The group is very concerned about socio-economic imbalances between Eastern and Western European countries, which can lead to a potential for economic exploitation specifically in the sex industry. This could have disastrous consequences in Eastern Europe as have been seen earlier in other parts of the world.

References

1. Centers for Disease Control. HIV/AIDS surveillance: US AIDS cases reported through November 1990. Atlanta: CDC, 1991.

2. Tyrrell R (unpublished). Strategies for reaching migrants and travellers - country report. London: Department of Health AIDS Unit, 1990.

3. Louhenapessy M. Rapport sur la prevention du SIDA pur les populations migrants en Belgique. Brussels: Service Social des Etrangers, 1990.

4. Haour-Knipe M. Assessing AIDS prevention: migrant populations. Paper presented at Assessing AIDS Prevention conference, Montreux, October 1990.

5. Gilmore N, Orkin A J, Duckett M, Grover S A. International travel and AIDS. Life Paths 1990; **2(2)**: 1-11.

6. De Schrijver A, Meheus A. International travel and sexually transmitted diseases. World Health Statistics Quarterly 1989; **42**: 90-99.

7. Van Duifhuizen R (unpublished). AIDS prevention towards migrants in the Netherlands - country report. Amsterdam: National Committee on AIDS Control, 1990.

Bibliography

Entzinger H B. Het minderhedenbeleid. Dilemmas voor de overheid in Nederland en zes andere immigratielanden in Europa. Boom: Meppel, 1984.

De la Cancela V. Minority AIDS prevention: moving beyond cultural perspectives towards sociopolitical empowerment. AIDS Education and Prevention 1989; **2**: 141-153.

Hendriks A, van Duifhuizen R. Report of the "Strategies towards migrants" workshops. Amsterdam: National Committee on AIDS Control, 1990.

Hendriks A. AIDS and Mobility. EUR/CP/GPA 023. Copenhagen: WHO Regional Office for Europe, 1991.

Organisation for Economic Co-operation and Development (OECD). Directorate for Social Affairs, Manpower and Education. SOPEMI: continuous reporting system on migration, 1989. Paris: OECD, 1990.

Schinke S P et al. African-American and Hispanic-American adolescents, HIV infection and preventive intervention. AIDS Education and Prevention 1990; **2**: 305-312.

Sleutjes M. Promoting safer sex among ethnic minority people: lifting the real barriers. *In:* Paalman M (ed). Promoting Sexual Health. Amsterdam/Lisse: Swets & Zeitlinger, 1990.

19

Opinion Formers

Background paper and report by Julian Meldrum, National AIDS Trust, London

Other members of the group were:

Norbert Gilmore (Chairperson)	*Canada*
Michael Bailey	*UK*
Hilary Curtis	*UK*
Fred Deven	*Belgium*
Elena Kabakchieva	*Bulgaria*
Patrick McGrath	*Ireland*
Nick Partridge	*UK*
Jos Poelman	*The Netherlands*
Lisa Power	*UK*
Ivo Procházka	*Czechoslovakia*
Therese Stutz Geiger	*Switzerland*
Barbara Suligoi	*Italy*
Kjell-Olav Svendsen	*Norway*
Liz Thornton	*UK*
Carmel Turner	*UK*
Lynne Walsh	*UK*

When we talk of opinion formers, what kind of opinions are we talking about — opinions shaping public policy, or opinions shaping private behaviour? Whose opinions — those of people with considerable power, or those of people who are powerless and at increased risk of illness and disability because of their lack of power — are we most concerned with? What weight should we give in health promotion to the personal health decisions of individuals, couples or dyads, compared to public policy decisions and norms within the groups shaping the society in which we live? Whose sexual health most needs promoting?

Who or what is an opinion former? Is there a distinction to be made between an activist — one who raises questions — and a more passive kind of opinion former, who persuasively suggests answers to other people's questions? If so, how can an opinion former be turned into an activist; how can an activist gain the status of an opinion former? And how can the negative influence of an activist or opinion former who is obstructing a programme be most effectively countered?

What is the message? How and when should HIV/AIDS issues be broadened or integrated with other issues? Should we be more concerned with the promotion of specific messages or with creating a climate of opinion? How do we deal in this context with genuine uncertainties and changing information?

This chapter raises many more questions than answers. But some broad conclusions may be stated at the outset. Some people do have, at times, a disproportionate influence over events and attitudes among audiences that health promotion workers seek to address. Such people must be identified and worked with to secure the success of health promotion programmes. This involves identifying, understanding, developing and exploiting connections with those who have power in society as it is now or is likely to become in the near future. Such a strategy carries risks as well as benefits, both for any campaign and for those opinion formers who become identified with it. Only by understanding these factors and working to develop and exploit opinion formers can their influence be maximised as a positive force in support of health promotion.

The Social Framework

The idea of "opinion formers" must arise from a model of how people form and maintain opinions and attitudes which affect health-related behaviour or the development of public policy. (In practice, campaigns which use mass media can and do shape private attitudes as well as public policy.)

If we are to discuss activism, we might ask whether activism directed at local and immediate concerns is different in nature and in strategies to be adopted from that which is directed at national or international and long-term concerns.

In relation to sexual health, a model of opinion formation could include:

1. Information and advice obtained through the mass media — identifying *media workers* as opinion formers, together with those most quoted in the media on issues of public concern, including *national or local politicians, public officials,* and *medical and other experts,* who are also *policy makers* in their own right. *Campaigners/lobbyists and interest groups* who seek to influence policy makers and the public at large may also fall into any of these categories, or into those which follow.

2. Information and advice obtained through personal contact with others considered to have special expertise — identifying *medical practitioners, health advisers* and other *advice workers* as key opinion formers. The discussion of the role of primary healthcare in promoting sexual health elsewhere in this report addresses the possibilities and limitations of working with some of these people.

3. Information obtained through formal education systems, identifying *schoolteachers, school governors,* and *college lecturers* as key opinion formers. This, too, is discussed elsewhere in this report, in relation to young people as an audience for health promotion.

4. Discussion and checking the significance of information received with people whose views and experience are valued — a wide category, which may include *parents, colleagues,* and *community and religious leaders,* some of whom gain status through formal institutions (eg. churches, trade unions) and some informally (eg. hairdressers, bar staff, "popular people", family elders).

What is the Message?

The medium, the message and the messenger cannot be discussed in isolation.

Does it make sense to attempt to address issues of HIV/AIDS and other sexually transmitted diseases together: are the messages to be conveyed the same or fundamentally different? Some of the earliest US and UK publicity on AIDS, in 1982 and 1983, seriously confused the public by placing the discussion in the context of scares about herpes. This may be a very good reason for directing some complex messages exclusively to interested and educated groups of opinion formers, especially professionals, rather than trying to make them *directly* accessible to the general public through wider campaigns.

Times have changed. It is hard to get any attention for sexually transmitted diseases other than HIV. While health education workers have approached employers asking about their HIV/AIDS policies, the idea of approaching employers to ask how they propose to promote the sexual health of their workforce is dismissed as ludicrous by UK health education workers. *But is this a situation that we should accept, or should we seek to promote wider awareness of the morbidity caused by STDs other than HIV?*

An alternative viewpoint is that we should be talking not of specific messages but of seeking to establish a broad climate of opinion, ie a supportive environment, within which health promotion workers will be free to direct the specific messages to people at most immediate risk of infection without provoking undue controversy, opposition or counter-productive effects. *Or is controversy healthy and to be courted?*

Examples of some of the possible messages are as follows:

Broad messages

- Sexual health is an important aspect of public health which needs to be treated seriously, funded adequately and not regarded as a political football;
- Promotion of sexual health is most likely to be effective if people are enabled to discuss sexual practices openly and rationally, without having moral values which they do not share imposed upon them;
- Discrimination, stigmatisation — anything which creates a "them and us" attitude — is unjust and likely to be counterproductive in public health terms. The enemy is the infection, not the person.

Messages which are specific but are relevant to any STD

- This STD should be a concern for everyone who is sexually active, and can not safely be dismissed as a problem for some other group of people. It doesn't go away when it isn't in the news.
- Safer sex is not always and not equally protective against all infections; condom users who have multiple or open relationships should continue to attend clinics.

Messages specific to non-HIV STDs

- There is a vaccine available against hepatitis B and anyone who might be at risk through their sexual lifestyle should seek testing and, if necessary, vaccination now.
- Most STDs can and should be treated as early as possible; they may be present without obvious symptoms, yet still cause serious problems.

Messages which relate HIV to other aspects of sexual health

- Different methods of contraception are associated with varying risks of HIV transmission and other STDs.
- Non-penetrative sex is not "deviant" and may, for some people, be entirely satisfying without carrying the risk of HIV transmission.

Examples of potentially confusing messages which relate HIV and other STDs:

- Untreated STDs increase the likelihood of HIV transmission; control of other STDs is therefore an important preventive measure in HIV/AIDS. HIV/AIDS control programmes must not be developed at the expense of other services to control STDs.
- Women who are HIV positive and who have been sexually active may be at higher risk of cervical cancer than other women, and should have more regular and thorough check-ups.
- Hepatitis B is more infectious than HIV; even those gay men, injecting drug users and health care workers who are strongly committed to safer sex and safe use of needles and other sharp instruments should still seek hepatitis B vaccination.
- Kaposi's sarcoma appears to be due to a sexually transmissible agent, which shows the need for people with HIV to practise safer sex even with others who are infected.

Working with the Mass Media

The print and broadcast media have given much space to stories on HIV and AIDS, and their response has been much studied and written about.

In Britain, the record of the broadcast media has generally been much better than that of the most widely circulated print media. In the USA, some print journalists (notably Lawrence Altman for the *New York Times*, Randy Shilts for the *San Francisco Chronicle*) have sustained AIDS assignments for periods of years. In Britain, such commitment has largely been confined to specialist magazines (*New Scientist*, *New Statesman and Society*, and the gay press, notably *Capital Gay*, *Gay Times* and the *Pink Paper*).

AIDS has changed the climate of opinion in British broadcasting, with increased acceptance on the part of the public and broadcasters that formerly taboo subjects can and must be aired. National television series made by and for gay men and lesbian women (Channel 4's *Out on Tuesday*) have been broadcast for the first time. A landmark series of discussions and films on sexuality was broadcast (Channel 4's *Sex Talk*), though many of the more personal contributions were familiar from other, earlier, documentaries only one of two of which have been suppressed (notably a 1986 BBC *Horizon* documentary on gay male sexuality and AIDS). Advertising of condoms is now allowed — though until very recently they could not be shown unrolled!

The media information work of well-established voluntary organisations and the development of professional public relations strategies by statutory health education agencies are probably of equal importance. For example, the UK Health Education Authority ran a television campaign early in 1990 which featured experts talking about the reality of heterosexual transmission of HIV, intended to counter versions of Michael Fumento's mistaken thesis (*The Myth of Heterosexual AIDS*) which were circulating among media workers. The campaign had an unexpected impact on a wider public, who found it clearer than previous campaigns. A further challenge on the same issue was made by the BMA Foundation for AIDS, taking the largest-circulation daily newspaper, *The Sun*, to the Press Council (a voluntary industry body concerned with press standards) and securing a judgment against the paper's announcement that "Straight sex cannot give you AIDS — Official".

The recent inclusion of a major story line on HIV in a popular English TV drama serial, *Eastenders,* has probably had as much impact as many paid-for advertisements. This was achieved as result both of the personal interest and commitment of members of the cast and production team and of the efforts of the Terrence Higgins Trust, which was itself featured in the programme.

Working with Politicians and Public Officials

Great effort has been directed at persuading politicians and public officials to recognise and acknowledge the nature and scale of the AIDS problem. Politicians themselves, such as Sir Norman Fowler when he was UK Secretary for Health and Social Security, and public officials such as the Chief Medical Officer Sir Donald Acheson, have played key roles in mobilising society to address the issue. In the USA, the impact of Surgeon-General Everett Koop's call for action, condom use and earlier sex education of youth was heightened by his track record as a conservative appointee of a conservative President.

In addition to the work of lobbyists from voluntary organisations, trade unions, professional bodies and industry, the work of parliamentary bodies such as the US Congressional Office of Technology Assessment and the UK Select Committee on Social Services has been of the greatest importance in identifying the public policy issues raised by AIDS and placing them on the political agenda.

The development in the UK of the All-Party Parliamentary Group on AIDS has provided a forum and channel for information — giving campaigners in voluntary organisations slightly increased access to politicians — which could be a model for international development in the European Community and/or the Council of Europe.

In contrast, however, almost no work was done in Britain until very recently (and then by voluntary organisations) on promoting vaccination against hepatitis B to those at most risk of sexual transmission. Universal vaccination — which may prove necessary if, for example, targetted campaigns fail to reach adolescents reluctant to face openly the implications of their possible future sexual behaviour — is not yet anywhere on the UK political agenda.

Working with "Medical Experts"

Some workers in any field of human activity come to greater public attention than others. In relation to AIDS, certain scientists and doctors have been seen as experts from very early in the epidemic and have been approached innumerable times to comment on all aspects of the problem. In some cases, this was at least initially due to formal positions of authority, in others to the particular skills of those individuals in presenting themselves and the issues clearly and vividly to the public. The same processes can be seen in relation to many other medical specialities, and have been deliberately fostered through schemes to identify experts willing to be quoted on a wide range of scientific and medical issues, for the benefit of journalists. The point to be considered is how and whether such individuals can or should be briefed and supported to prevent spurious impressions of expert disagreement being created from what are merely differing emphases, or from people being drawn into commenting on issues beyond their own expertise. The WHO Global Programme on AIDS has intervened in this area with a series of consensus statements seeking to establish expert perspectives on what can be seen as "morally contentious" issues. *How effective and useful have these statements been?*

Working with Professional Groups and Specialist Advisers

The UK Department of Health devoted considerable effort to circulating all doctors with information on AIDS, early in the course of its first awareness campaign, presumably reflecting the role of doctors in transmitting information and shaping opinions.

The record of the gateway medical journals, such as the *New England Journal of Medicine, Lancet, British Medical Journal*, among others, in making space for AIDS reports, has been excellent from the first recognition of AIDS. It continues to be the case that a substantial proportion of major research papers on HIV and AIDS are published in widely-read journals.

Training in HIV counselling has been a priority within the NHS response to AIDS, with the establishment of the National AIDS Counselling Training Units, the Learning About AIDS Project at Bristol Polytechnic, and additionally a great deal of work by voluntary agencies such as the Terrence Higgins Trust.

The BMA Foundation for AIDS is, in itself, a direct response by leading members of a professional body to the need for health education and policy initiatives which have credibility with their members.

Working with Community Leaders

Selectively targetting this broadest category of "opinion formers" may not always be possible through the mass media, but a style of campaign which encourages people to get the facts and to discuss them with others could still be founded on recognition of their importance. At its most basic, a campaign directed at parents, giving advice on what they should tell their children or grand-children, would fall into this category; this approach has of course been taken in relation to cigarettes and alcohol. *Is this approach transferable to a subject which parents may be more reluctant to discuss with their children?*

The use of "workshop approaches" does open up the possibility of recruiting and training peer-group educators among adults in a range of settings. The work of Janet St Lawrence and Jeff Kelly, based at the University of Mississippi, has become deservedly famous — using a diffusion model for information, recruiting popular individuals as agents of change in Mississippi gay bars. But other examples of the same processes in action can be seen in many places: for example, in a prison, many things can be conveyed to prison staff for more effectively by a well-briefed and respected prison officer than by any outsider. Distance learning techniques might be employed to educate such educators, involving very specialised use of mass media.

Community Development

Health promotion aimed at identifying and mobilising community leaders raises wider questions of the value and place of community development. Certainly, the response of gay communities — real or imaginary, unified or diverse — has been considerable, and the sense of a supportive community has often grown with the response to AIDS. *This process has its limits — what are they?*

Amsterdam is exceptional in its Junkie Unions for drug users — elsewhere, the sense of community among drug users may be more difficult to establish. Other "communities" which have been forced to respond to AIDS include universities, ethnic minorities (eg. the Haitian community in Montreal), and people with disabilities — obviously families affected by haemophilia but also, in Britain, profoundly deaf people who rely on sign-language for communication, who have suffered disproportionately from HIV disease.

As Simon Watney and others have argued, the idea of a "heterosexual community" is problematic. However, there are many other expressions of community, such as around sports teams, which could and in some places already have been harnessed to safer sex messages, for example, Liverpool Health Promotion Unit's work with Liverpool Football Club.

The development of a supportive community of people with AIDS and HIV has been of great importance in enabling individuals to share their own experience with a wider public and contribute actively to the debate on all aspects of HIV and AIDS, which has had a major impact on opinion formers.

How is Effectiveness to be Measured?

Surveys of public opinion, monitoring of media coverage, and assessment of the rationality and coherence of policies adopted could all be taken as measures of the effectiveness of campaigns directed at opinion formers.

To identify the impact of any specific campaign will be difficult and almost pointless, unless the campaign in question is focussed on novel and very precise messages. The essence of working with opinion formers is to seek to reinforce efforts to communicate that are proceeding through a range of different channels at any one time. When the multiplier effect begins to appear — when new organisations and individuals take up the challenge of responding to HIV/AIDS and other threats to sexual and public health, the benefit is obvious.

20

Primary Health Care and Sexual Health Promotion

Report by Peter Anderson (author of background paper), Primary Health Care Unit, Churchill Hospital, Oxford, with Jan Kristoffersen (chairperson), Skårer Health Centre, Skårer, Norway

Other members of the group were:

Maria Albota	*Germany*
Dénes Bánhegyi	*Hungary*
Hanspeter Bosshard	*Switzerland*
Pat Evans	*UK*
Susanne Flyborg	*Sweden*
Christine Godfrey	*UK*
Judith Gosmore	*UK*
Joan Holmes	*UK*
Hilary Hughes	*UK*
Gregory Lucas	*UK*
Airi Poder	*Estonia*
Mary Russell	*Ireland*
Svein Steinert	*Norway*
Ronald Valdiserri	*USA*
Derek Williams	*UK*

Introduction

The working group approached its task with the recognition that the context of primary health care varies in different countries, and that the topic of primary health care had not been addressed in the previous workshop. Thus the group sought to develop recommendations which were widely applicable and which individuals could take back to their own countries and expand upon in more detail.

The group took the view that integration of HIV/STD prevention and sexual health promotion activities is important and in many ways is easier to undertake in primary care settings, where providers are used to dealing with individuals in relationships and with individuals in families, rather than with separate conditions or diseases. The advantages and disadvantages of integrating sexual health promotion into general health promotion should be carefully assessed, and may depend on the strength of the existing framework of preventive and health promotion activities and services. In many countries the pre-existing skills among primary health care workers represent an important potential resource for promoting sexual health. We now have some understanding of determinants of health-related behaviour and the stages and processes which individuals go through in trying to change their behaviour, and thus there are advantages in considering the commonalities of different behaviours, be they sexual, eating or substance use behaviours. For these reasons, this chapter considers general aspects of health promotion in primary health care settings as well as the specific features applicable to sexual health.

Towards a Sexual Health Strategy

The World Health Organisation committed itself to the goals for *Health For All by the year 2000* in 1977[1] and, with the declaration of Alma-Ata on Primary Health Care in 1978, recognised the importance of primary health care as a means of achieving health for all[2].

The member states of the European region of the World Health Organisation have agreed that in order to improve health in Europe, efforts should be concentrated on the reduction or elimination of preventable diseases, the promotion of healthy lifestyles and the provision of comprehensive health coverage for the whole population, based on primary health care, with particular attention being given to vulnerable or at risk groups in society[3]. As part of the Health For All strategy a set of 38 targets was formulated by the European Region of WHO, and these can be broken down into 3 sub-sets:

- targets for improvements in health (reducing or eliminating preventable conditions or reducing mortality);

- targets for activities needed to bring about improvements in lifestyle, (eg. reducing tobacco consumption, alcohol and drug use, reducing environmental health risks and improving the environment);

- targets designed to improve the management and organisation of health services, the quality of care and the training of health workers.

The WHO Division of Noncommunicable Diseases encourages an integrated approach to prevention and control activities[4]. The basic principle is that diseases with common causes (unhealthy lifestyles and deficiencies in preventive services) should be approached with a common strategy of health promotion and provision of preventive health services. The prevention of HIV transmission involves promoting changes in lifestyles, and thus might be integrated into an overall effort to influence positive health behaviours.

The implementation of a health strategy is a shared responsibility with activity at least six levels, which include:

Individuals

The individual is both the starting point and the target of a health strategy. Through the many roles that individuals fulfil in their daily lives, they are afforded numerous opportunities for promoting health and preventing disease. With these opportunities, however, comes personal responsibility. Measurable decreases in risks to health can result from individual changes in diet, exercise, tobacco use, alcohol use and sexual habits. However, while the responsibility for change lies with individuals it also lies with society and individuals cannot be expected to act alone.

The family

The family is the primary context in which health promotion activities occur and is therefore potentially the most immediate source of health-related support and sex education for the individual. It is in the context of the family that attitudes and behaviours regarding diet, physical activity, smoking, alcohol use and sexual activity are often learned and maintained. Thus, the family offers the primary opportunity for change in many areas of health-related behaviour.

However, the potential of the family in promoting sexual health has not been well explored, and there is a need to appreciate the specific religious and cultural issues surrounding sex and sexuality. For example it may not be realistic to expect families to discuss highly sensitive issues such as detailed sexual behaviour and HIV/STD prevention. It is also unclear how the influence of the family compares to that of, say, peer groups in shaping individual attitudes and perceptions.

Individuals with less socially accepted social orientations, eg homosexuality, may be even more deprived of family support in developing a healthy sexual lifestyle.

In any event, the family should not be expected to assume responsibility for fostering healthy behavioural patterns in isolation. Families require the support of communities in achieving and maintaining good health. This is particularly important in areas of deprivation.

Communities

Community based health programmes play a strong role in improving the health status of families and individuals. Multiple opportunities exist for community health promotion efforts on the part of government, voluntary and non-statutory groups, industry and education services. Local community programmes are often more efficient than centralised programmes managed far away from the point of delivery. Indigenous programmes maintain the sensitivity to the family and neighbourhood values that is vital to encourage change, successfully, towards healthier lifestyles within the community.

Health professionals

For many, primary health care professionals are the primary sources of health information. Sexual health is unusual in this respect, in that information has been widely distributed through mass media or other channels while hitherto the role of professionals may have been under-used. Professional training gives health professionals the skill to translate science into practice. Practice can take the form of partnerships with non-professionals in pursuit of individuals', families' and communities' health care. The effectiveness and efficiency of sexual health promotion services will be enhanced by such partnerships.

Sexual health education and counselling in particular provide opportunities for interdisciplinary and intersectoral work in order to integrate health practices into the daily lives of individuals, their families and communities. Professional associations can facilitate dissemination of the health promotion and disease prevention knowledge-base through their established information exchange and professional education networks. A special opportunity and responsibility exists for the teachers of health professionals to equip them with expertise and skills to share their knowledge with the public.

Primary Health Care and the Implementation of a Health Strategy

Primary health care providers have a key role in supporting individuals, families and communities in a sexual health strategy. For the purposes of this chapter, primary health care providers include general practitioners, primary health care nurses (practice nurses, community nurses and public health nurses), reception and administrative staff, although some might argue that open-access community family planning and STD clinics also fall within the definition of primary health care.

There is extensive research data to support the role of primary health care providers in supporting individual lifestyle change, particularly smoking cessation, reduction in alcohol use amd non-pharmacological intervention to lower elevated blood pressure and thus reduce coronary morbidity and mortality.

Sexual health

There have been few studies, however, examining the effectiveness of primary care providers in influencing sexual behaviour of patients[5]. Clearly the effectiveness of counselling will depend on the age, level of maturity, sex, parity, and health history of the patient as well as on the level of training, clinical practice setting and counselling skills of the provider.

Studies of clinic-based educational programmes for the prevention of HIV infection and other STDs, which in some cases have included physician counselling as a component, have reported increased rates of return for test of cure and reduced incidence of certain STDs. However, these studies involved only certain populations and provided little evidence of change in sexual behaviour[5].

In terms of prevention of unintended pregnancy the effectiveness of counselling has been studied primarily in the context of sex education in schools and family planning clinics. No studies have been undertaken investigating the effectiveness of physician or nurse advice on condom usage.

For effective use of resources in sexual health promotion, there is a need to identify key target audiences to be reached, for example adolescents, injecting drug users, gay men etc. Greater information is needed on how these populations interact with existing primary care services, and how services can be made more user-friendly for them.

Impediments to implementation

Although there are sound clinical reasons for emphasising prevention in the primary health care setting, studies have shown that primary care providers often fail to provide clinical preventive services[5]. This can be due to a variety of factors including lack of reimbursement. Also busy practitioners often have insufficient time with patients to deliver the range of preventive services that are recommended. But even when these barriers to implementation are accounted for, primary care providers fail to perform preventive services as recommended. One reason for this is uncertainty among physicians as to which services should be offered.

Part of the uncertainty derives from the fact that recommendations come from multiple sources and these recommendations are often different. In addition a major reason why primary care providers may be reluctant to perform preventive services is scepticism about their clinical effectiveness. It is often unclear whether performance of certain preventive interventions can significantly reduce morbidity or mortality from the target condition one is attempting to prevent. It is also unclear how to compare the relative effectiveness of different preventive services, making it difficult for busy practitioners to decide which interventions are most important during a brief patient visit. A broader concern may be that some interventions could result in more harm than good. A specific concern in sexual health is understanding concepts about sexual health[6,7] and having the skills for sexual health counselling.

There is thus a need to develop means of evaluating the impact and quality of sexual health promotion in primary health care. Such evaluation should look not only at quantitative data, but also the quality of sexual health promotion services offered by primary health care providers to their clients. Based upon such evaluation, it is then important to develop nationally agreed comprehensive recommendations addressing clinical preventive services and to provide support and education in implementing these services.

The role of primary health care in supporting environmental change

The definition of health promotion used by the WHO Regional Office for Europe is: "Health Promotion is the process enabling individuals and communities to increase control over the determinants of health and thereby improve their health"[8].

The Alma-Ata report stated that health promotion seeks to enable individuals and communities to increase control over the determinants of health and thereby improve their health. It is therefore concerned not only with enabling the development of lifestyles and individual competence to influence factors determining health, but also with community intervention to reinforce factors supporting healthy lifestyles and to change those factors preventing or prohibiting healthy lifestyles.

It would seem legitimate for primary health care teams to take an interest in the health environment and seek to influence it, while at the same time promoting appropriate personal health behaviour by individuals and families. At present many primary health care providers give personal advice to patients as the opportunity arises during routine patient-initiated consultations, and this can be seen as an attempt to influence both personal health behaviour and the general health environment. A multidisciplinary team is more likely to be able to carry out broad-based health promotion activities than individual isolated practitioners. The skills of primary health care nurses, including public health nurses, are invaluable in local action focussing on the health environment.

Examples of Initiatives to Encourage Health Promotion in Primary Care Settings

The 1990 general practice contract

A new contract for general medical practices has been introduced in the United Kingdom which recognises the importance of primary health care as a means to support a health strategy[9,10,11]. The contract was based on the evidence that immunisations and screening tests are important preventive services. However, the most promising role for prevention in current medical practice now lies in changing the personal health behaviours of individuals long before clinical disease develops.

One of the requirements of the new contract is to offer all newly registered patients a "health check", which should include ascertainment of factors in the patient's lifestyle which may affect his or her health. A similar health check must also be offered to all registered patients aged 16-74 years who have not been seen within the preceding three years. These checks may be an occasion on which to offer sexual health promotion, particularly to young healthy adults who might not otherwise be in contact with services.

The new contract has also introduced a system of payments for preventive services. Thus GPs are eligible for payments if more than a certain percentage of registered women patients aged 25-64 undergo cervical smear testing, and can be paid fees for providing health promotion clinics. There is scope for further development of such clinics to provide targetted health promotion including sexual health.

Finally, a new allowance is paid to GPs who participate in approved post-graduate education covering three subject areas: health promotion and prevention of illness; disease management; and service management. This new financial incentive appears to have been a major boost to post-graduate education.

The role of facilitators and supporters

In the UK and The Netherlands facilitator programmes have been set up to enable and support organisational change within the general practice including setting up of risk management programmes, the adoption of minimum standards for screening and intervention, and audit of records. Facilitators have been shown to lead to an increased recording of risk factors in patient notes[12]. Intervention practices with facilitator support recorded twice as much blood pressure, four times as much smoking and five times as much weight as control practices without facilitator support. In the UK, facilitators have been also been appointed for the prevention of HIV infection[13].

Supporting Implementation

The role of primary health care providers in sexual health promotion initiatives can be summarised under the headings used in the Ottawa Charter for Health Promotion — enabling, mediating and advocacy. The challenge is for primary health care providers to look beyond the confines of the one-to-one consultation or even of family care, and to accept that their role is to work with others to enable the community as a whole to increase its control over the determinants of health. Primary health care teams need to deal with local issues but they can also join with other workers to initiate and support regional and national health promotion initiatives.

One implication of the move from disease prevention to health promotion is the need for intersectoral collaboration. Collaboration may take place at a number of levels. District levels are probably the most important in terms of the organisation and administration of primary health care, since these tend to deal with policy issues and can most easily liaise with local authorities. However, collaboration also needs to take place at a local practice level between both non-statutory and statutory agencies.

To promote effective multisectoral working, national AIDS programmes need to continue both to deliver specific targetted services and to provide support and education to primary health care. In both disease prevention and health promotion activity, it is important to determine the boundaries of the work primary health care providers can be involved in and when they may need to involve other organisations and services.

At present many education and training curricula for primary health care providers neglect health promotion and disease prevention, sexual health issues and counselling skills. Continuing professional education should specifically deal with the management of health promotion projects with skills, including those required for collaboration of other professions and with the problems of implementation of health promotion programmes.

A particular area for development is in supporting adolescent health care, both in terms of service provision and the general health environment, since primary health care services have sometimes been poor in meeting the needs of adolescents. Creating a user-friendly environment includes removing practical obstacles such as cost and availability of services, condoms, and other contraceptives.

Provision of guidelines

One of the reasons for failure of primary care providers to provide recommended services is a lack of nationally agreed clinical guidelines as to which services should be offered. It is important therefore, to produce guidelines for preventive and sexual health promotion services[14]. Such guidelines are needed for the individual and family support role of primary care services and for their role in supporting community health promotion programmes.

Relevant issues for individual and family support include the initiation, maintenance and changing of behavioural patterns; and the influence of sources of stress and social support on attitudes and behaviour. Issues to be covered in guidelines for community activities include how to involve people and encourage their participation; assessment of communities to determine health problems and coping resources; defining measurable objectives for health outcomes, risk factors, levels of awareness, service availability and use, and levels of protection achieved, and monitoring progress towards these objectives; and development of interventions which are comprehensive, multi-faceted and culturally relevant.

Materials

Clinical interventions have been demonstrated to be more effective when supported by the provision of self-help materials. The use of self-help materials enables empowerment of patients and shift in the locus of control to the patient. Appropriate materials can also provide protocols for clinical interventions which lead to increased compliance and increased quality. There is room for further development of appropriate resources for use in promoting sexual health in the primary health care context, for example sexual health packs to support increased uptake of screening services and increased use of condoms.

Training

The provision of guidelines and resources will support a training programme in prevention and health promotion that needs to be provided at the levels of basic professional education, vocational training and continuing education. Training and ongoing follow-up contact can encourage general practitioners to participate in health promotion activities. In a blood pressure education project, it was found that patients of doctors who had attended a single tutorial achieved lower blood pressures than patients of doctors who had not[15]. General practitioners who undergo training including smoking cessation activities have higher patient-abstinence rates after 1 year than those who do not receive training[16]. Follow-up contact reinforces training about lifestyle interventions. Thus ongoing support after a training workshop produced general utilisation rates for smoking cessation programmes of 84% at 6 months, compared with 57% for no follow-up contact.

Education and training needs to support primary health care providers in supporting individuals, families and communities undertaking and maintaining behaviour change. Education and training needs to cover the principles and processes of behavioural change and counselling techniques to support this.

Somatic, emotional, intellectual and social aspects of human sexuality should be components of basic professional training and education for primary health care providers. Continuing education in sexual health promotion should be developed based upon assessment of need and incorporated into existing frameworks where possible. Experience suggests that multi-disciplinary training and education is important in this context, as are allowing providers time out from their work to reflect and providing on-going contact and support.

Education needs to cover the management of health promotion projects with skills, especially those required for collaboration of other professionals and with the problems of implementation of prevention and health promotion programmes.

Dissemination and networking

The prevention and health promotion knowledge base needs to be disseminated through established professional information exchange systems and professional education networks.

Demonstration projects must be accurately described and evaluated, so that others can learn from their successes and failures. It is important therefore, to have effective networking so that primary health care providers can be informed of health promotion projects being undertaken elsewhere.

Conclusion

Primary health care is an important setting for sexual health promotion activities, and is particularly suited to integration of STD/HIV prevention with other aspects of sexual health, since primary health care providers are used to dealing with individuals in relationships and individuals in families rather than with separate conditions or diseases. Assessment of client's health status should routinely include a sexual health dimension, recognising both the importance of human sexuality to individual health and the importance of a person's health status to their sexuality. Primary health care services should be made more user-friendly, especially for adolescents, and this includes removing practical obstacles such as cost and availability of condoms, contraceptives and the services themselves. Multi-disciplinary and inter-sectoral approaches should be developed within the framework of primary health care to deal more effectively with health promotion.

References

1. World Health Organisation. Global Strategy for Health for All by the year 2000. Geneva: World Health Organisation, 1981.

2. World Health Organisation. Primary health care. Geneva: World Health Organisation, 1978.

3. World Health Organisation Regional Office for Europe. Targets for Health for All. Targets in support of the European Regional Strategy for Health for All. Copenhagen: WHO, 1985.

4. Interhealth Steering Committee. Demonstration projects for the integrated prevention and control of non-communicable diseases. World Health Statistics Quarterly, 1991; **44**: 48-54.

5. US Preventative Services Task Force. Guide to clinical preventative services. Baltimore: Williams and Wilkins, 1989.

6. World Health Organisation Regional Office for Europe. Concepts for sexual health. EUR/ICP/MCH 521. Copenhagen: WHO, 1986.

7. World Health Organisation Regional Office for Europe. Sexuality and family planning. Copenhagen: WHO, 1986.

8. World Health Organisation Regional Office for Europe. The role of primary health care in changing lifestyles. Copenhagen: WHO, 1989.

9. Department of Health. General practice in the National Health Service. A New Contract. London: Department of Health, 1989.

10. Department of Health. Terms of service for doctors in general practice. London: Department of Health, 1990.

11. Department of Health. Statement of fees and allowances payable to General Medical Practitioners in England and Wales from 1st April 1990. London: Department of Health, 1990.

12. Fullard E, Fowler G, Gray M. Facilitating prevention in primary care. Br Med J 1984; **289**: 1585-87.

13. Mayon-White R, Kirsch G, Anderson P. An integrated response to HIV and AIDS in Oxfordshire. *In* Pye M, Kapila M, Buckley G, Cunningham D (eds). Responding to the AIDS challenge. London: Health Education Authority, 1989.

14. Anderson P. HIV and sexually transmitted diseases. *In* Fowler G, Gray J A M, Anderson P (Eds). Preventive medicine in general practice. 2nd ed. Oxford: Oxford University Press, *in press*.

15. Inui T S, Yourtee E L, Williamson J W. Improved outcomes in hypertension after physician tutorials: a controlled trial. Ann Int Med 1976; **84**: 646-651.

16. Richmond R L, Anderson P. Lessons from conducting research into general practice for smokers and excessive drinkers; the experience in Australia and the United Kingdom. Submitted for publication, 1991.

21

The Political and Legislative Framework in which Sexual Health Promotion Takes Place

Background paper and report by Aart Hendriks, Gay and Lesbian Studies Department, University of Utrecht, and Dutch National Committee on AIDS Control

Other working group members were:

Julia Häusermann (Chairperson)	*UK*
Laura Ayres	*Portugal*
James Barrett	*UK*
Denis Bridoux	*UK*
Ailsa Butler	*UK*
Peggy Clarke	*USA*
Rosmarie Erben	*WHO*
Robin Gorna	*EC/Luxembourg/UK*
Bent Hansen	*Denmark*
Judith Hilton	*UK*
Naomi Honigsbaum	*UK*
Peter Jackson	*UK*
Henning Jørgensen	*Denmark*
Mukesh Kapila	*UK*
Sue Lucas	*UK*
Peter Makara	*Hungary*
José Manshanden	*The Netherlands*
Ilie Marcu	*Romania*
Lindsay Neil	*UK*
Airi Poder	*Estonia*
Henriette Roscam Abbing	*The Netherlands*
Bertino Somaini	*Switzerland*
Kåre Tönnesen	*Norway*

"If one cannot legitimately seek sensuous pleasure in sexual experience, then the arousal and gratification of sensuous desires cannot be an embodiment of a virtuous love"

Susan T. Nicholson, Sinful sex.[*]

Introduction

Health and disease are of the utmost importance for individuals and society as a whole. Promoting health, including sexual health, and preventing disease have been societal objectives throughout human history. These objectives have been transformed into concrete policies, directed at bringing about particular changes or results[1].

---

[*] In: The Journal of Religious Ethics, as quoted in Pierce C, Van De Veer D (eds). AIDS, ethics and public policy. Belmont, CA: Wadsworth Publishing Company, 1988.

Health and disease are complex phenomena that need to be considered in their wider societal perspective. There is general consensus that health and disease prevalence inter-relate strongly with social and economic conditions. Health promotion and prevention of diseases are interwoven with the entire social, economic and political fabric of a country. In principle, health promotion and disease prevention measures are most likely to work if they go hand in hand with long-term improvement in social and economic conditions for the population at large[2], and hence promoting sexual health and preventing sexually transmittable diseases should form part of overall policy to improve standards of living.

Unlike disease prevention policies, there has so far been little academic analysis of comprehensive and cohesive policy to promote sexual health. Mostly, health policies have been reactive, responding to symptoms considered to threaten the health of individuals or society as a whole. There are good reasons to believe that health policies should instead be proactive, anticipatory and holistic in approach.

Ten years after AIDS was first documented, many notions on how best to contain sexually transmitted diseases (STDs) have completely changed. It sounds grotesque, but thanks to HIV/AIDS we now have a far better, though still inadequate, knowledge of human sexuality and the internal and external influences on its expression. The present HIV/AIDS epidemic, and steeply rising global incidence of certain STDs with similar transmission routes, urge us to evaluate health promotion models currently in use and in particular to assess how far they are appropriate to sexual health.

This chapter reflects the outcome of eight hours of discussion on how to construct an accurate political and legislative framework for promoting sexual health that fulfills the needs of our time. In accordance with the discussions in the working group and the structure of the background paper[3], this article focuses on the determinants and general principles of (sexual) health policy. Special attention will be paid to the legal and ethical aspects of promoting sexual health. Though the outlook of this article is primarily European, it is believed that its conclusions and recommendations are of importance to the world community as a whole.

What is Sexual Health?

Before we can discuss how best to promote sexual health, we first need a clear concept of what we understand by sexual health. Several definitions of health have been put forward in the past, that have inspired us to develop a working definition of sexual health.

Narrowly defined, health can mean a state of absence of disease and pain. But the World Health Organization (WHO) has opted for a broader definition, describing health as "a state of complete physical, mental and social well-being, and not merely the absence of disease or infirmity"[4]. A conference on the right to health care, held under the auspices of the United Nations University, adopted the following definition: "Health is a state in which one does not feel the body ... When you offer men and women health, you let them have the freedom of their body, the freedom of their movements. However modest it may be, the freedom of one's body is already the beginning of one's freedom."[5]

Similarly it can be maintained that sexual health means more than avoidance of diseases and pain caused by sex. In 1974 WHO defined sexual health as "the integration of the physical, emotional, intellectual and social aspects of sexual being, in ways that are enriching and that enhance personality, communication and love".* We chose the following definition: "*Sexual health is an integral part of overall health, not restricted to the avoidance of STDs and HIV/AIDS. Sexual health contributes to the fulfillment of individual sexuality, enabling a person to share this with consenting others, without jeopardizing the health and well-being of other persons. Sexual health requires the enjoyment of free choice, expression and responsibility, with particular regard to the prevention of transmission of STDs/HIV. The sexual health of an individual contributes to the well-being and health of the individual involved, his/her sexual partner(s), and the ultimate community as a whole*".

These definitions of health and sexual health emphasize that the right to individual self-determination is a prerequisite for enjoyment of (sexual) health. According to Dr Svein-Erik Ekeid, European regional co-ordinator of WHO's Global Programme on AIDS, only a person who says "yes" to sexuality has the strength to say "no" to risky sexual behaviour (see page 17). At the same time, it should be stressed that the individual's right to self-

---

* Quoted in AIDSAction, Issue 13. London: AHRTAG, 1991.

determination is not unlimited. As with many human rights, it may need to be balanced against the rights of others. This does not imply that individual and community interests are automatically in opposition. Most often the rights of the individual and public health interests of the community are in a direct line and reinforce each other, with the one flowing from the other (see below)[6].

Promoting Sexual Health

Simply stated, health promotion comprises all efforts to protect, maintain and improve health. Health promotion thus encompasses actions relating both to the health of the individual and to general conditions affecting the public health of society as a whole[7]. Health promotion, being an issue of the whole community, needs to be clearly distinguished from disease prevention, which is mainly a field for medical specialists. Health promotion presupposes a relationship of trust between those who undertake actions to promote health and the recipients of these activities. Health promotion activities can only succeed if the members of the target group are willing and able to learn and benefit from the provided means. This usually implies the full participation of representatives of the target group in the process of developing and implementing a health policy.

The guiding principles for developing effective health policies were formulated at the first International Conference on Health Promotion in Ottawa, Canada, and include:

- Building healthy public policies;
- Creating supportive environments;
- Strengthening community skills;
- Developing personal skills: and
- Reorienting services.*

It follows that when designing a health policy, three levels of action should be distinguished:

- Individual-oriented health promotion as it takes place at home, at school, etc.
- Community-oriented health promotion to reach people both as individuals and as members of a social group.
- Environment-oriented health promotion such as measures related to safe food, safe water, safe blood, etc[2].

Promoting sexual health is a special form of health promotion, and follows the same levels of action. The principles laid down in the Ottawa Declaration are fully applicable. There are, however, a number of obstacles to be aware of which may impede effective implementation of sexual health programmes. Barriers to overcome include:

- Misconceptions such as the notion that sex is solely a procreational activity (see page 8) or that only adults have sex.
- Taboos which impede discussing sexuality in general or specific forms of sexuality.
- Use of incomprehensible and unclear language.

Promoting sexual health in the context of STDs and HIV/AIDS poses additional hindrances. As noted above, health promotion presupposes a relationship of trust between providers and recipients of health promotion activities. In case of HIV/AIDS and a number of other STDs, we are confronted with a situation in which these diseases disproportionally affect individuals whose lifestyles many people find objectable. As a result, people with HIV/AIDS or STDs, their partners and carers, and others associated with these diseases become stigmatized and discriminated against[8]. Stigmatization and discrimination not only mean a flagrant violation of some of the fundamental rights of the persons concerned, but also undermine the efforts made by health promotion workers[9]. In this respect Wendy E. Parmet described discrimination as "a cruel and painful accomplice of STDs and HIV/AIDS, that moreover weakens our ability to limit their spread"[10].

---

* Ottawa Declaration. Final document of the First International Conference on Health Promotion, Ottawa, Canada, 21 November 1986.

The Policy Makers

The promotion of health, including of sexual health, requires adequate structures for design and implemenation of policies and allocation of sufficient resources. As an issue affecting the whole community, health promotion demands the involvement of all community groups and cannot, in the words of a Latina AIDS activist living in New York, "be imposed by one group on another. The only way to do [it] is to respect, support and utilize the strengths, talents and potentials for change in each country's racial and ethnic [and other — AH] communities"[11].

At present, an overview of HIV/AIDS policy making bodies shows wide disparity as to their composition, representativeness, and decision making powers. At one extreme there are bodies exclusively composed of members with a (bio)medical background, while at the other extreme there are bodies with a broad, interdisciplinary composition. The decision making bodies tend to have in common that they are predominantly white and male[3].

To be effective and to develop socially acceptable policies, (sexual) health promotion bodies should be functional, powerful, multidisciplinary, and participatory, particularly on the part of affected community groups. Due attention should be paid to the effective co-ordination of policies and activities being developed and implemented by the various bodies, at the national, sub-national and international levels (see below).

The Subjects of a Sexual Health Policy

A sexual health policy can only succeed in achieving the goals set out above, as long as an integral, cohesive approach is adopted based on public health principles and human rights law. Such a policy should be geared to the distinct needs of the various groups in society, taking into account age, gender, sexual orientation, socio-cultural norms, etc. As noted above, a sexual health policy should be directed concurrently towards individuals, communities and the environment.

Environment-oriented measures affect the population as a whole and should primarily enable people to enjoy healthy sexual lifestyles, independent of their sex and sexual orientation. Such measures may include quality standards for condoms, the provision of accurate and correct sexual health information, etc.

Concerning individuals and communities, policy makers have to acknowledge that people differ in many respects, including their sexual behaviour, sexual fantasies and sexual identities. The sexual lifestyle an individual adopts depends to a considerable extent on his or her interactions with the community, notably his or her peer group, which explains the potential key role of these groups in promoting sexual health.

The fact that people are not created equally becomes particularly manifest when addressing health issues, including sexual health. We are not only different with regard to our attributes, capabilities and good fortune[7], but especially our susceptibility to diseases, our immunological resistance and psychological potential to cope effectively with internal and external demands[12]. Moreover, we are people of different sexes with individual sexual preferences as to with whom and how we most enjoy having sex. Respecting sexual pluralism, both on an individual and a community level, is the basis for a sound sexual health policy.

Thus, a sexual health policy both aims at reaching individuals and communities, and is directed towards creating the necessary environmental conditions for enjoying sexual health. By doing so, policy makers may need to pay special attention to people with special needs, children, and vulnerable members of society, in order to guarantee that these persons as well can fully enjoy the right of each human being to sexuality and to share sex with other consenting adults.

Policy Strategies and Models

Successful sexual health promotion is likely to form part of an overall policy to improve health and to prevent diseases, which would include social measures such as improving the standard of living, guaranteeing a decent income for all members of society and high quality nutrition.

158

Given the limitations of sexual health promotion, there is an undeniable need for better understanding of how to formulate a sexual health policy, especially in view of the prevalence of STDs which may undermine its goals. Historically, public health strategies related to sexual health and reducing the spread of STDs have included:

- Education and counselling;
- Case finding;
- Treatment and patient care;
- Notification;
- Epidemiological surveillance; and
- Regulatory measures[13].

From these strategies it is immediately clear that traditionally emphasis has been on disease control and prevention, with few policy instruments developed to promote sexual health. This can partly be explained by the strong impact of the host-agent-environment model of disease causation[2]. As its name already suggests, this model is purely epidemiological in nature and almost completely neglects non-medical factors influencing people's health and well-being. Despite the development of health promotion as an independent discipline, medical professionals have always had a strong influence on the formulation of sexual health strategies. This can best be illustrated by referring to the different health models underlying the organisation and co-ordination of primary HIV/AIDS prevention at the national level. In grouping national responses within Europe, Hans Moerkerk distinguished four different models[14]:

1)   Countries with a *pragmatic response*. This group embraces the countries where AIDS/HIV prevention policy is defined on the basis of facts and overall consensus, resulting in straightforward, outspoken and non-discriminatory campaigns. These countries first formulated their HIV/AIDS policies at the start of the HIV/AIDS epidemic (1983-84), and adopted policies emphasising information and education. Moreover, information and education methods became carefully geared to the needs of the various population groups. Voluntary behavioural changes and the prevention of negative reactions were given priority above prohibition and coercive forms of control. Mid-term and long-term strategies were set out, and regularly evaluated. Close involvement and room for manoeuvre of non-governmental organizations (NGOs) and AIDS service organizations (ASOs) are another characteristic of the health model adopted by these countries.

2)   Countries with a *political response*. This refers to the countries where the contents of the HIV/AIDS prevention policy are mainly determined by what is politically possible as well as desirable. Since national policy makers see the law as an appropriate instrument to regulate and possibly to modify human behaviour, large numbers of legal amendments and new legislation have been endorsed. Governments only seem willing to collaborate with NGOs and ASOs as long as these share the same goals.

3)   Countries with a *bio-medical response*. In these countries HIV/AIDS is mainly regarded as a medical issue. It is held that HIV/AIDS can best be contained by giving bio-medical professionals full responsibility for formulation of policy. Consequently, bio-medical specialists dominate all HIV/AIDS policy making bodies and are scarcely accountable to non-medical or independent bodies. While Governments have displayed only short-term interest in the issue, NGOs and ASOs are either non-existent or completely neglected by the policy making institutions.

4)   Countries with an *emergent response*. This category embraces the countries where HIV/AIDS has only recently been identified as a serious public health concern. An adequate HIV/AIDS prevention policy has as yet to be formulated. Existing legislation is used as the basis for HIV/AIDS control. Networks of NGOs and ASOs, if they exist at all, are poorly developed.

On examining HIV/AIDS and sexual health policy making in the various European countries, it has to be concluded that these four models apply not only to HIV/AIDS prevention but to the entire process of national sexual health policy making. One clarification can be made with reference to the category of emergent responses. Within this group of countries (Moerkerk particularly thought of the central and eastern European countries) there are countries leaning more or less towards a pragmatic response, e.g. Czechoslovakia, Estonia, Hungary, Latvia and Slovenia. Other countries, eg Lithuania, Russia and Poland, appear to adopt a political response, while Bulgaria has the characteristics of developing a bio-medical response.

There are also European countries that so far cannot be said to have formulated an HIV/AIDS prevention and sexual health policy, such as Romania, Albania and some former Soviet republics. The designation *retarded response*, indicating that there is barely a coherent prevention, care and research strategy, let alone a sexual health policy, is probably most appropriate to describe the current state of affairs[3].

The Role of the Law

There is a crucial role for the law in designing a sexual health policy. Legislation reflects the fundamental values of society and constitutes a means to guarantee enjoyment of these values. The law not only defines the tasks and duties of the State, it also describes the limits of its authority and the procedures the State and its agents are bound to follow when performing their tasks. Besides the relationship between the State and its citizens, the law can regulate the relations between private individuals and their relation towards the physical environment. Moreover, the law is a means to balance (potentially) opposing interests.

Legislation also sets the general framework of action in the area of health care, including the promotion of sexual health. In this respect it is important to bear in mind that the law is instrumental and never an aim in itself[15].

The basis for State action in the field of sexual health is encompassed in the right to health care. The right to health care can be defined as the right of all individual citizens to share the benefits of health care and health services in society, which should be of a high quality, geographically accessible and financially affordable. Following its nature as a social and economic right, the right to health care is primarily an obligation on States to provide sufficient means to guarantee its citizens a (minimum-indispensable) standard of health, as well as equal access to health services. At the same time this right draws attention to the individual's responsibility[16,17,18].

For the formulation of a sexual health policy, a number of rights and principles have to be observed vis-à-vis State action. While sometimes considered as limitations, these rights and principles guarantee the just and appropriate exercise of State authority in the interest of all. Rights that govern State action in the area of sexual health include:

- The *right to privacy**, reflecting the idea that an individual should be protected against any undue interference with his/her private space and autonomy. In addition to the protection of one's family, home and correspondence, the right to privacy, as embodied in the international treaties, also protects the individual's particular identity, integrity, intimacy, autonomy, private communication and sexuality[19]. The right to privacy is also the legal basis of the right to individual self-determination, the doctrine of informed consent and the principle of confidentiality[18];

- The *right to life*[†], enshrining guarantees against intentional deprivation of life;

- The *prohibition of torture, maltreatment and improper medical experimentation*[‡], protecting individuals from certain forms of cruel and unusual treatment. Moreover, this right may impose a duty on the State to guarantee certain standards in institutions that are directly under its supervision, like prisons[20]; and

- The *right not to be discriminated against***, reflecting the idea that all persons are equal as concerning their dignity[7]. This right also implies that health care should be made equally accessible to all people and that special efforts should be made to redress health inequalities[18].

Besides these obligations, all enshrined in human rights law, to be duly respected by the policy makers, there are

---

* Art. 12, Universal Declaration of Human Rights (UDHR); Art. 17, International Covenant on Civil and Political Rights (CCPR); Art. 8, European Convention on Human Rights (ECHR).

† Art. 3, UDHR; Art. 6, CCPR; Art. 2 ECHR.

‡ Art. 5 UDHR, Art. 7 CCPR; Art.3 ECHR; Art 5, Convention Against Torture; Preamble to European Convention for the Prevention of Torture.

** Art. 2, UDHR; Art. 2, 26, CCPR; Art. 14, ECHR; Art.2 International Convention on Social, Economic and Cultural Rights; Preamble to WHO Constitution; Preamble to European Social Charter.

a number of guiding principles of utmost importance when developing a policy to promote sexual health.

- *Equality of treatment.* All people should be treated equally before the law and public regulations, regardless of the population group to which they belong or their individual characteristics;

- *Relevance.* Public action should be clearly geared to the problem at hand;

- *Proportionality.* Limitations of individual freedom imposed by public action must be no greater than is commensurate with the benefit and objectives they achieve;

- *Effectiveness.* Measures must be adequate and appropriate to bring about particular changes or results;

- *Feasibility.* Each measure should be implementable in the real world, given social, economic, cultural and political circumstances and constraints; and

- *Ethical acceptability.* In general measures should be acceptable to the concerned community, and in particular, should respect the ethical principles of autonomy, beneficence, non-maleficence and justice[15,21].

The law also provides rules for policy makers on how to balance different interests at issue. Very few rights are absolute in nature, and where rights conflict they need to be carefully balanced.

In promoting sexual health, the State can choose between a broad array of approaches. At one extreme, the State can attempt fully to empower and enable individuals and communities to attain knowledge, attitudes, believes and practices that are to the benefit of the sexual life and sexual well-being of all. Alternatively, the State can take absolute responsibility for the sexual health and sexual well-being of all members of society. From a legal perspective, the first approach would imply strengthening the rights of individuals, encouraging them voluntarily to adopt behavioural changes where necessary, though not automatically imply neglect of the individual's responsibility towards others. The second approach would favour increased interference on the part of the State in the private life of individual citizens, through measures regulating and prescribing private and public conduct.

To determine which approach is best, one should look at both human rights law and the principles above. These imply that a sexual health policy should not only be in accordance with the (human rights) law, but should be relevant, proportional, effective, feasible, ethically acceptable and should guarantee equality of treatment. An international consultation on legislation, ethics and HIV/AIDS recommended in this respect that health legislation should be used in a positive way to promote and support health education and distribution of information to provide the public with the means for voluntary behaviour change. The consequent policy corresponds more with the first approach above than with the second[15].

Besides measures directed towards individuals and communities, legislation enables (and obliges) the State to introduce measures to promote conditions in which the population as a whole can enjoy healthy sexual life and sexual well-being. Such measures may include condom advocacy campaigns — though some States still presume that this would incite "promiscuity" — controlling the quality of health care instruments, screening donor blood, etc. It goes without saying that such environment-oriented measures should be in accordance with the law and the guiding principles above.

In conclusion, the law plays a supportive role in promoting sexual health. Abelin defined health-oriented legislation as legislation intended to support health promotion, based on the recognition of health as a highly valued priority[2]. Review of health legislation in many countries, particularly in the field of infectious diseases, shows, however, that many regulations have become irrelevant, out-dated or even counter-productive[22]. Thus an international consultation recommended that health legislation be regularly re-evaluated, and inefficient regulations repealed[15].

Determinants and General Principles of a Sexual Health Policy

In paying due attention to the individual, community and environment levels for sexual health promotion measures, it is obvious that each requires its own institutional infrastructure, specialized personnel and technical support. However, measures need to be carefully integrated for the cohesiveness of the overall policy.

The working group identified the following five determinants:

- STDs/HIV transmission has to be prevented through correct, non-judgmental, understandable and targetted information and education;

- Legislation should be used in a supportive way, to promote voluntary responsible behaviour, fully respecting human rights law;

- Special attention should be paid to the (sexual health) needs of vulnerable people, notably members of socially and culturally marginalized population groups;

- Discrimination and stigmatization on the basis of (presumed) health status should be effectively prevented, and countered where it exists;

- Representatives of the target groups should participate in all phases of designing and implementing the policy.

General principles include that:

- All health policy should be defined in the light of (individual and social) human rights and ethics. Moreover, measures need to have a public health rationale. The principles of autonomy, integrity, individual self-determination and the rights to privacy, informed consent, secrecy, access to medical records, access to medical care and freedom from discrimination are of key importance.

- As with general health, society is best protected from outbreaks of (sexually transmissible) diseases by safeguarding individual human rights and empowering and enabling the individual to make healthy choices the easiest choices, as concerns sexual life and sexual well-being.

- Policy making should be participatory and multi-disciplinary. There should be an identifiable co-ordinating body, whether a government, ministry or committee, specially entrusted to develop sexual health policies. It should be given the necessary powers to ensure effective implementation of the policies developed.

- The Ottawa Declaration is fully applicable when defining a sexual health policy.

- A sexual health policy should safeguard the rights and integrity of vulnerable people, particularly those who (are forced to) engage in non-consensual sex and/or are unable to express their own free will.

- Sexual health policies should be defined in the light of known scientific facts, should respond to identifiable needs and avoid being moralistic or judgmental.

- Due attention should be paid to the diverse forms of human sexuality, recognizing that policies must include people with special needs as well as sexual, ethnic and other minorities.

- Equal access to social benefits, and the adequate funding of these, are pre-conditions for fulfillment of sexual health. Making access to social benefits dependent on the person's sexual lifestyle, or route of transmission of a STD or HIV, contradicts human right law and undermines sexual health.

- The professional codes of people working in the (para-)medical sector should be in conformity with human rights law.

- The law is an important, but not the sole tool in achieving overall (sexual) health. The legislator has ultimate responsibility for ensuring that these determinants and principles operate, and are seen to do so.

International Issues

Policies to promote sexual health and prevent STDs/HIV have an impact far beyond national borders. This holds true particularly for Europe, where the process of European integration and the falling away of artificial, almost insurmountable borders have produced unprecedented stimuli for travel and migration. Modern means of transport, notably air traffic, facilitate this phenomenon[23].

From previous research it is known that international mobility is an important though generally underestimated epidemiological component, because people who are "away from home" or living in an alien socio-cultural environment are apparently less empowered and/or enabled to make healthy (sexual) choices. Though entrance restrictions may seem an efficient means to deny entrance to national territories to people with communicable diseases, where STDs or HIV/AIDS are concerned such restrictions are ineffective, unjustified and disproportionate. At best and at great cost, they only briefly retard the spread of STDs and HIV infection[24,25,26,27].

Instead, innovative methods have to be developed to promote sexual health at the cross-boundary level. There should at least be close collaboration between institutions and individuals working in sexual health promotion in different countries. Concerted action should be considered to empower internationally mobile people to protect their sexual health and that of others, without stigma or discrimination[23].

Furthermore, there should be an attempt at reaching international agreement on what is and is not safer sex (and safer drug use). Distinct health messages in different countries have been proven to undermine efforts optimally to inform people about sexual health[23].

Other issues affecting the efficiency of sexual health campaigns that may need international attention are:

- Access to health care services for aliens;
- Treatment of non-nationals with STDs or HIV/AIDS;
- Access to clinical trials and drugs;
- Access to condoms, needles and syringes;
- International quality standards for condoms;
- Sexual exploitation as a result of economic imbalances between people and countries (in Europe notably between East and West), and
- Avoidance of discrimination on the basis of health status, in both vertical and horizontal relations.

As at national and local levels, adequate international and regional structures are needed to develop and implement clear, cohesive sexual health policies which reach as many people as possible.

Recommendations

The working group agreed a number of recommendations, without suggesting that these are comprehensive. Those recommendations headed "General" were produced by the group as a whole, while the others were developed by smaller sub-groups working under the respective titles.

General

- There should be a dynamic analysis of the effectiveness of sexual health policies, so counter-productive policies can be avoided and removed;

- Sexuality should be portrayed positively, not restricted to a means of procreation;

- Sexual health policies should be adequately resourced so individuals actually receive the services and support they require;

- Social benefits related to sexual health, and risk reducing equipment (e.g. condoms) should not only be easily and equally accessible, but also affordable;

- Segregation, isolation and discrimination on the basis of sexual health or lifestyle are counterproductive and undermine the goals of promoting sexual health: and

- Homosexuality, prostitution and purchase of sexual services should be decriminalized and destigmatized.

Surveillance, detection and reporting

- The practice of voluntary testing, based upon informed consent and embedded in a range of services, should be upheld;

- Only in exceptional cases should the principle of medical confidentiality and the right not to know of HIV/STD infection be bypassed; and

- Special provisions are needed for minors, people with special needs and those unable to express their own free will, to benefit from these principles.

Education, information, counselling

- Education should aim to empower individuals to make free choices on the basis of adequate information;

- Correct, non-judgmental and understandable information, education and counselling should be provided sufficiently, geared to the specific needs of various population groups;

- Sex education should be organized in both formal and non-formal settings;

- It should aim at assisting the individual to develop the necessary skills to benefit from freedom of choice, correctly assessing health risks to him/herself and others;

- It should include information about STDs and HIV/AIDS, but not be restricted thereto; and

- Travel and immigration restrictions are not justifiable as a means to prevent spread of STDs and HIV/AIDS, and testing incoming people is ineffective, unjustified, disproportional, costly and harmful. Instead, innovative education and information methods should be developed to empower internationally mobile people to protect their sexual health and that of others.

Development of a supportive environment

- Development of solidarity, tolerance and non-stigmatization is fundamental to a supportive environment;

- Sexual health policies should be supported by an appropriate legal and ethical framework;

- They should be supported by the development of environments which empower people to make their own free choices in relation to sexual health and sexuality.

- International standards should be developed to ensure high quality of condoms.

- Since sex and drugs issues cannot be wholly separated, particularly in the context of STDs/HIV/AIDS, there should be integrated provision of needles, syringes and methadone with sexual health services;

- Due attention must be paid to ensure that policies implemented in penitentiary and other closed institutions take full account of these principles. Moreover, health care services in such institutions should be provided independently of the security system;

- The war on drugs should end, since it is a war on drug users and alienates them from the communities in which they live, impeding the effectiveness of (sexual) health promotion and harm reduction strategies;

- A code of conduct for researchers is urgently needed, reflecting their societal responsibility;

- Legislation and supportive procedures should protect against sexual harassment, abuse and rape, including rape in marriage;

- Legislation should prevent unauthorized recording of personal information relating to HIV/STDs and/or sexual lifestyle where this serves no legitimate aim and may undermine public health;

- Legislation should guarantee equal treatment and prohibit discrimination on grounds of race, gender, sexual orientation, disability, health status, needs and other considerations; and

- Legislation should be regularly re-evaluated to ensure it is up-to-date. Where necessary, laws should be amended, removed or added.

Conclusions

Promoting sexual health is an essential element of general health promotion and disease prevention. It is an issue for the whole community, not just for medical professionals. Sexual health policies need to be re-evaluated regularly on the basis of up-to-date information and the fullest possible understanding of sex, sexuality, STDs/HIV and the social factors influencing sexual and social behaviour. In this respect, sexual health must be defined in broad terms, not merely as the absence of (sexually transmitted) disease and pain.

A sexual health policy starts with the policy makers, definition of aims, identification of target groups and development of an integrated strategy. A number of determinants and general principles underlie all sexual health policies. In this respect the law is instrumental, not an aim in itself.

In addition to construction of a framework for developing a sexual health policy, this article recommends various concrete measures for formulating and implementing such a policy.

Although the working group was primarily concerned with the national context for policy making, we acknowledged fully that promoting sexual health has an impact that goes beyond national borders. It is crucially important that international dimensions of sexual health promotion receive more attention in the near future and that adequate international and regional structures be established for design and implementation of clear, cohesive sexual health policies.

References

1. Kapila M. The prevention of AIDS and other STDs: issues for policy makers. *In* Paalman M (ed). Promoting Safer Sex. Amsterdam/Lisse: Swets & Zeitlinger, 1990.

2. Abelin T. Approaches to health promotion and disease prevention. *In* Abelin T, Brzezinski Z J, Carstairs V D L (eds). Measurement in health promotion and protection. WHO Regional Publications, European Series No. 22. Copenhagen: WHO Regional Office for Europe, 1987.

3. Hendriks A. What can we learn from 10 years AIDS policy making? *In* Background papers and transcript of closing plenary session of the Second International Workshop on Preventing the Sexual Transmission of HIV and other STDs, Cambridge, 24-27 March 1991 (Report). London: BMA Foundation for AIDS, 1991.

4. World Health Organisation. Preamble to WHO Constitution, Official Records No. 2, June 1948.

5. Dupuy R-J (ed). Le droit à la santé en tant que droit de l'homme (The right to health as a human right). Workshop, The Hague, 27-29 July 1978. Alphen aan den Rijn: Sijthoff & Noordhoff, 1979.

6. Parmet W. Legal rights and communicable disease: AIDS, the police power and individual liberty. Journal of Health Politics, Policy and Law 1989; **14**: 741-771.

7. Pan-American Health Organisation (PAHO). The right to health in the Americas: a comparative constitutional study. PAHO Scientific Publications No. 509. Washington, DC: PAHO, 1989.

8. Tomasevski K. AIDS and human rights. *In* IMADR Yearbook 1989, Vol. 2. Tokyo: International Movement Against all forms of Discrimination and Racism, 1990.

9. Carlé P, Hendriks A, Zeegers D. AIDS and human rights in the European Communities. Zoetermeer: Dutch National Council for Public Health, December 1990.

10. Parmet W. An anti-discrimination law: necessary but not sufficient. *In* Gostin L O (ed). AIDS and the Health Care System. New Haven/London: Yale University Press, 1990.

11. Rodriguez R. We have the expertise, we need resources. *In* The ActUP/NY - Women and AIDS Book Group. Women, AIDS and Activism. Boston: South End Press, 1991.

12. Noack H. Concepts of health and health promotion. *In* Abelin T, Brzezinski Z J, Carstairs V D L (eds). Measurement in health promotion and protection. WHO Regional Publications, European Series No. 22. Copenhagen: WHO Regional Office for Europe, 1987.

13. Intergovernmental Committee on AIDS (IGCA) Legal Working Party. Legislative approaches to public health control of HIV-infection. Canberra: Department of Community Services and Health, 1991.

14. Moerkerk H. AIDS prevention strategies in European countries. *In* Paalman M (ed). Promoting Safer Sex. Amsterdam/Lisse: Swets & Zeitlinger, 1990.

15. Directorate of Health. Health legislation and ethics in the field of AIDS and HIV infection. Report on an international consultation, Oslo, 26-29 April 1988. Oslo: Helsedirektoratet (Directorate of Health), 1989.

16. Roscam Abbing H D C. International organisations in Europe and the right to health care. Deventer: Kluwer, 1979.

17. Leenen H J J, Roscam Abbing H D C. Bestuurlijk gezondheidsrecht. Alphen aan den Rijn/Brussels: Samson H D Tjeenk Willink, 1986.

18. Hendriks A, Nowak M. The impact of advanced methods of medical treatment on human rights. *In* Weeramantry C G (ed). Science, technology and human rights: some case studies. Tokyo: United Nations University, 1991.

19. Nowak M. UNO - Pakt über bürgerliche und politsche Rechte und Fakultativprotokoll - CCPR Kommentar. Kehl/Strasbourg/Arlington: N P Engel Publisher, 1989.

20. Neveloff Dubler N. Depriving prisoners of medical care: a "cruel and unusual" punishment. Hastings Center Report 1979; 9: 7-10.

21. Martin J. Health policy and the AIDS epidemic: the call for public health interventions: the use of legislation for prevention, its tasks and limits. Medicine and Law 1989; 8: 233-241.

22. Jean J P. Les problèmes juridiques soulevés par le développement des MST et leur prévention. *In* Job-Spira N, Moatti J P, Spencer B, Bouvet E (eds). Santé publique et maladies à transmission sexuelle. Paris/London: John Libbey Eurotext, 1990.

23. Hendriks A. AIDS and mobility (Report). Amsterdam: National Committee on AIDS Control, 1991.

24. Sommerville M A. The case against HIV antibody testing of refugees and immigrants. Canadian Medical Association Journal 1989; 141: 889-894.

25. Gilmore N, Orkin A J, Duckett M, Grover S A. International travel and AIDS. Life Paths 1990; 2 No.2: 1, 6-11.

26. Hendriks A. The right to freedom of movement and the (un)lawfulness of AIDS/HIV specific travel restrictions from a European perspective. Nordic Journal of International Law 1990; 59(2-3): 186-203.

27. Goethart R. Internationaal verkeer van personen en HIV-infectie. Report of Interuniversitair samenwerkingsverband Universiteit van Amsterdam, Instituut voor Sociale Geneeskunde, Sectie Gezondheidsrecht en Rijksuniversiteit Limburg, Vakgroep Gezondheidsrecht. Maastricht: Rijksuniversiteit Limburg, 1991.

22

Sex Work

*At the First International Workshop on Prevention of Sexual Transmission of AIDS and other STDs there was a working group on "Prostitutes and their clients", which produced the following conclusions and recommendations:**

- Prostitution arises from a demand for sexual services. It can only exist in the presence of clients and often third parties, who control the activities or benefit from them.
- Everyone who is engaged in prostitution should be aware of the risks of HIV/STD infection and supported in efforts to take adequate precautions.
- Prostitutes, themselves, are willing to take responsibility for safer sex very seriously, when given the opportunity to do so. In addition to prostitutes, other involved persons (clients and third parties who control the activities) should take responsibility for safer sex and be addressed with prevention activities.
- Members of the different target groups must be involved in the development and implementation of STD/AIDS prevention.
- Governments should support prevention activities by supplying the necessary human and financial resources.
- Anything that drives prostitution underground destructs, inhibits and interferes with attempts to promote safer sex.
- Governments should, therefore, examine the effectiveness of their laws regarding prostitution. If these laws are ineffective or even counterproductive for prevention activities, they should be altered or abolished (decriminalisation of prostitutes).
- Mandatory testing does not seem to be effective. The public health infrastructure should enable voluntary and accessible medical care.

During the Second International Workshop on Prevention of Sexual Transmission of AIDS and other STDs there was no working group specifically on sex work arranged by the organisers. However, a special unofficial working group on sex work met during the workshop and submitted this report, prepared by Ruth Morgan Thomas, Alcohol Research Group, Department of Psychiatry, University of Edinburgh:

We regret that sex work was not included as a separate issue at this workshop, particularly since the majority of plenary speakers have raised the issue of prostitution.

When we refer to the sex industry we are not only talking about male and female sex workers but about all other parties involved in commercial sex: for example clients, who research has shown outnumber sex workers by at least 50:1, and all other individuals who are involved in the control of prostitution such as brothel managers, pimps and law enforcement agencies. Too often people imagine that prostitution is something that prostitutes do on their own and amongst themselves. Given this common misunderstanding it is not difficult to understand why conference organisers so often focus on the sex workers in isolation. However it is essential that the sex industry is examined in a holistic context which acknowledges the involvement of numerous associated individuals and agencies *other* than sex workers. Given this fact it is essential that sex work is in future allocated an independent forum in which to explore the multi-faceted and complex issues associated with it, such as child prostitution, psychoactive drug use, migration and international trafficking of sex workers, and the effect of legal and judicial systems on harm minimization within the sex industry. Clearly we have not had adequate time or space to address the many issues around sex work which require urgent attention. However, we would wish to reaffirm the conclusions drawn at the first workshop and would reiterate the need for all legal, social, political and religious barriers to effective HIV prevention strategies to be removed.

---

* Biersteker S. Promoting safer sex in prostitution: impediments and opportunities. *In:* Paalman M (ed). Promoting safer sex. Amsterdam/Lisse: Swets & Zeitlinger, 1990.

Maria Paalman
Director,
Dutch Foundation for STD Control,
Utrecht

I hope you will acknowledge the difficulty I had in preparing this closing address. I had to be at all the meetings, which left little time actually to sit down and write. Often people who give closing addresses make it up beforehand. I didn't do that so I hope you will accept that it's not entirely well-structured and maybe some things could have been said better.

When the Dutch Foundation for STD Control organised the first meeting of this kind in Noordwijkerhout two years ago, our objectives were to invite people who were experts in their specific fields to be able to share their experiences, data and ideas. The format of that meeting, with a lot of time to discuss things, was regarded as so successful that the Health Education Authority in London was asked to take care of this second event. That first meeting was called Promoting Safer Sex. The British opted for Promoting Sexual Health to put safer sex in a wider context. But it should not lead us away from the key issues at stake.

Sex

We still tend to be a bit sheepish about sex. There are still countries that are trying to implement sex education in schools, for instance, without allowing people to speak freely about sex, let alone about different sexual techniques, condoms etc. I was very glad therefore, that Dr Svein-Erik Ekeid of WHO spoke out on the inherently positive experience that sex can be and very often is.

Coming from a background in STD and AIDS control, I can understand his concerns, and those of others involved in HIV education, about the moralising atmosphere of STD programmes in some countries. I also appreciate the differences between HIV and other STDs. But I do want to stand up for the many STD services that have managed to train their doctors, nurses and educators in non-judgemental communication with clients. The very fact that they work in STD control means that they have accepted the sexual behaviour that can potentially lead to an infection.

From a biological viewpoint it is argued that human beings are not monogamous by nature. Yet many programmes advocate monogamy. I wonder what makes politicians or decision makers think that they can achieve something that the Catholic Church, for instance, has not achieved after centuries of trying very hard.

Our goal can be neither to promote promiscuity nor to abolish it. It's a pointless battle. Instead of fighting windmills we should be pragmatic. It's a measure of our inconsistencies that the HEA vetoed the organisers' idea of distributing a condom to each participant. We are allowed to talk about condoms for three days, but beware that we should have one or worse use it.

Considering this, Section 28 on homosexuality, and the legal restrictions on depicting genitals in information and booklets, I am left wondering whether the UK is driving backwards into the future. Are we restaging the comedy of several decades ago, "No sex please, we're British"? I really hope not. In most European countries a lot has changed for the better in terms of openness about sexuality due to the AIDS epidemic. It would be sad if the British Isles feel that they do not yet belong to that Europe.

When we ourselves can be so hypocritical, how can we expect to convince our decision makers, let alone our target audiences, of the benefits of safer sex? How many of us have actually tried it? I think it would be a good thing in the next workshop if people would have the guts to sit down and discuss their own behaviour honestly with each other: to do a small non-representative sample of the difficulties. We are still not there in knowing why people have so many problems in changing the behaviour that could save their lives.

Compared to the results of the first workshop, did we get any further on the road to sexual health, or healthy sex? The answer is yes and no. One cannot expect much progress in less than two years in such a complicated area as influencing people's most private behaviour.

Over the past years I have continually voiced, and heard others voice, the need for more research on sexual behaviour its determinants in order to understand better why some people sometimes make healthy choices and others do not. I have not heard much news in that area, except a little bit in the working group on men who have sex with men, gay men, where there was discussion about the reasons for what epidemiologists call "relapse".

Integrating HIV Prevention, STD Control and Sexual Health Promotion

1. Possibly the greatest development over the last two years has taken place in the area of integrating HIV prevention into STD prevention, sex education, health promotion, primary health care and family planning. There was a working group on family planning, STDs, and reproductive health, and another on primary health care and community settings — both new from the first meeting. I think such integration is a very sound strategy in a time of declining resources for HIV prevention.

It is my firm belief that, in the long run, mainstreaming HIV education into general sexual health education is the only way to safeguard the positive results of the AIDS epidemic, more openness on sexuality issues, high quality behavioural research in some countries, and a vast reservoir of new expertise.

Nevertheless, there are reasons for caution in integrating STD in HIV information campaigns, especially mass media campaigns, and it is something we should go about very carefully. I even think it is not possible at the present time. One could perhaps have a campaign on viral diseases and focus on the fact that they cannot be cured. But the vast amount of information and differences between STDs — not just between HIV and other STDs — are too much to pile into one information campaign. But I do think that combined safe sex and condom campaigns are proper.

As was discussed in the working group for gay men and is also true for drug users, prostitutes and other marginalised groups in society, mainstreaming holds a danger of losing the expertise which has been built up in the fields of peer education and self-help. We should consider how to preserve the best of both worlds.

2. A new issue which has emerged is that safer sex behaviour for HIV is not always safe sex for other STDs. We need to find out more about this, because it must be a frustrating and demotivating experience to find one has contracted an STD while following the guidelines.

3. In many European countries estimates of HIV prevalence have been reduced over the past years. Although that was probably in part due to earlier over-estimates, there has been well-documented behaviour change which definitely contributed, and we should be very happy about that. There is a drawback, however, in that most people perceive their personal risk as being low, and policy makers may use the figures to cut prevention budgets. The very success of prevention programmes could kill them; such is the paradox of successful prevention. The same thing happened in the 50s and the 60s after the sharp decline in STDs following the wide-scale use of penicillin. There is a historical lesson here that should not be overlooked.

Challenges for the Future

Some of the new areas that have emerged during the Workshop which require further thought include:

- *Mainstreaming of health promotion activities implies training* — of many different groups: health workers, doctors, nurses, family planners, teachers, maybe even travel agents, many others. Training is needed not only in the technicalities of STDs and HIV but particularly about sexuality issues, and about effective and respectful communication, for instance on risk assessment and risk reduction behaviour.

- *The overlap between care and prevention has yet to be explored in full.* It is well known that mass media campaigns alone are not enough to change all people's behaviour. Many targetted activities have taken place for different population groups but, taking it a step further, there are possibilities for individual education in the form of counselling and support. The most relevant people for this expensive type of education are *people who are HIV positive and people seeking treatment for a suspected STD.* Those who are already infected are obviously the ones who can spread diseases, especially when there is no cure or no symptoms to alert them. For HIV positive people and people with AIDS, care, support, counselling and the buddy system offer possibilities for preventive education that have to be looked into more seriously. People who seek medical attention for a suspected STD are a self-selected sample from the general population who have had unsafe sex. The time when a person is most receptive to preventive counselling is when he or she is diagnosed with an actual STD. Both groups should be included in the next conference, because they are very important target groups.

- *Travel was another point that surfaced in different working groups:* the high mobility of injecting drug users in southern Europe; the well-documented mobility of sex workers. The subject has acquired a new impulse from the socio-economic changes in Eastern European countries, with women going into prostitution in the West. We should also be aware of men going for sex tourism to Thailand and other countries, young people on holiday, businessmen and of course conference attenders. With the open borders in 1992 and the opening up of the Eastern European countries, healthy travel seems to become a more and more important issue.

- *Alcohol use seems to be an important co-factor in unsafe sex.* There have been some conflicting reports in the past, but now there seems to be more evidence. The possibility of combining "safer drinking" and "safer sex" campaigns should be explored.

Many other issues came up in the working groups, including strategies for education, how to involve people from the target audiences themselves, social context issues, empowering people, privacy, confidentiality — it was all in there. I do not want to comment in detail, because all of these things have come up before and are covered in the proceedings of the last meeting. I do want to point out, though, that the *fact* that they keep coming up, in various fora, means that they have not been dealt with sufficiently, and cannot be dealt with quickly. It takes time, but it is proper and important to keep repeating them.

Points from the Working Group Reports

As I was listening to the reports from the different working groups, I noted a few things which I thought were new points, besides those already mentioned:

- Just about every working group struggled with definitions. It is important to get clarity amongst ourselves as to what we are talking about. I'm glad all groups did that and I hope it will be reflected in the proceedings.

- The next point was brought up in the primary health care group. As we start mainstreaming our activities and end up with a plethora of organisations working on sexual health, then we have to be clear about the limits and the boundaries of who is doing what.

- Someone from the condom working group said that it is not so easy to use a condom properly. It is true that you have to learn it, but after a few times it is as easy as putting on your socks. One wouldn't want people to go away with the idea that it is too difficult to learn how to use condoms.

- It is becoming steadily clearer that when implementing strategies for a given target audience one has to look at the differences within the audience, the sub-groups within groups.

- The media and political lobbying discussed in the opinion formers working group was a completely new field that we entered this time, and it was a very lively group with people debating on high levels. They came up with a lot of good questions, more than answers, but that only underlines the need to have a working group on that again and to see whether we can get any further.

Another important point I want to stress is the welcome tendency to see a person not only as someone having an STD or being HIV positive. Gay men have jobs, do something in their free time, prostitutes might have a child or follow a course in French. Looking at the whole context of people's lives is important.

There are some further points for the organiser of the next meeting to note. There should be a working group on men who have sex with women; on prostitutes; on travellers. In fact, those three were suggested, all of them, for this meeting. Commercial sex workers were combined with women in general during this meeting, but the other two were left out for reasons of space. All would be good choices for next time.

There has been very good attendance at the workshop, with about two hundred people from twenty-eight countries including twenty-two people from *Eastern European countries*. It was a wise decision of the HEA to make it possible for the people from Eastern Europe to come. We do have a problem there. A gap in knowledge, and maybe also in attitudes, was apparent between the Western and Eastern countries on the whole issue of promoting sexual health, which was there for historical reasons. In saying this I do not intend to discriminate, but am merely stating a fact. The Eastern countries need to learn fast, so it was very good that they could come here and I hope they have learned a lot. It would be a good idea for WHO Europe to carry that further and make haste in organising training workshops, where we could share our experience with them in a more structured manner and help them decide what they could do in their own countries.

The last point I want to close with because it is the most encompassing one which concerns the whole theme of this workshop. That was the call for a *model sexual health policy* on a national level. I think that the HEA in London, having a five year programme on sexual health, should probably take this idea and try to develop such a model.

Finally, this conference has been a serious one, a lot of serious things have been discussed. I'm delighted that in spite of that we also had fun together. Many of us have been in this field for a long time and we have to protect ourselves from burning out. Humour is a good way to get new energy. Thank you all for the supportive atmosphere.

This summary is based upon the conclusions and recommendations of the various working groups as presented to the closing plenary session of the workshop. However, some groups have included more detailed conclusions and recommendations in their written reports elsewhere in this book. After the workshop the organisers circulated a booklet containing the summary to individuals and organisations with an interest in promotion of sexual health. The text was as follows:

Recommendations of the Second International Workshop on Preventing the Sexual Transmission of HIV and other Sexually Transmitted Diseases, Cambridge 24-27 March 1991

This paper summarises the recommendations and conclusions of a multidisciplinary workshop organised by the UK Health Education Authority and the British Medical Association Foundation for AIDS, co-sponsored by the World Health Organisation and held under the auspices of Mrs Catherine Lalumiere, Secretary General of the Council of Europe*. The 200 invited experts who participated in the workshop included health promotion and health education specialists from statutory and voluntary sector agencies and academic institutions. The workshop focussed especially on sexual health promotion within the European context, with most participants coming from this region, including countries of central and Eastern Europe.

The organisers of the workshop have compiled together these recommendations and are circulating them widely to promote their implementation. The full proceedings of the workshop will be published at a later date.

Recommendations relating to the political and legislative framework in which sexual health promotion takes place

Adequate structures are required at the international, national and local levels in order for clear, cohesive sexual health policies to be developed and implemented. At national level, there should be an identifiable coordinating body, whether a government ministry or national committee, specifically entrusted to develop sexual health policies. Such a body should be required to cooperate with all other relevant ministries, bodies and organisations. It should be given the necessary power and resources to ensure effective implementation of policy.

Experience with AIDS has confirmed that, far from there being a conflict between the enjoyment of individual rights on the one hand and societal interests on the other, *respect for individual rights and dignity is an essential component of effective sexual health policies.* Other essential such components include the following:

> they should be based on sound scientific knowledge;
> they should be developed in response to identifiable needs;
> there should be dynamic analysis of their effectiveness, so that counter-productive policies, such as coercive laws, can be avoided and removed;
> they should avoid moralistic or judgemental attitudes, stigmatisation and discrimination;
> they must be supported by appropriate legal and ethical frameworks;
> they should foster development of a supportive environment which empowers people to make their own choices in relation to sexual health;
> they should be adequately resourced so that individuals actually receive the services and support they

---

* The recommendations contained in this document are of the workshop participants and do not necessarily represent the views of the organising or co-sponsoring bodies.

require.

The most effective policies are those based upon informed consent, and which are participatory and voluntary, rather than coercive.

The sponsors of the Promoting Sexual Health workshop should support a group to develop a model sexual health policy which recognises the right of all people to express their sexuality positively in fulfilling and satisfying ways without abusing the rights of others. This policy should be relevant to all, but with a particular reference to the unassailable right of young people to become sexually aware, to prevent unplanned pregnancies, transmission of HIV and other STDs, and to receive clear and accurate information which is non-judgemental, from educators experienced and trained in this field. It should take into account confidentiality, free and informed choice, free and easy access to a range of alternative services, sex education in schools, required funding, and national and local structures to support its implementation.

There should be active participation of all relevant sectors of society in sexual health policy making including, in particular, women, minorities including sexual minorities, people with special needs and those directly affected by the policies. In the context of AIDS, people infected with HIV should participate in policy making.

Legislation should guarantee equal treatment and prohibit discrimination on grounds of race, gender, sexual orientation, disability, health status, needs and other considerations. Equal access to health care and other services should be ensured and should not depend on sexual lifestyle or the route of acquisition of an STD.

Legislation should be introduced to prevent unauthorised recording of personal information relating to HIV/STDs and/or sexual lifestyle where this does not serve a legitimate purpose.

Travel and immigration restrictions are not justifiable as a measure to prevent STDs, and mandatory testing for incoming people is impractical, ineffective, costly and harmful.

Legislation and supportive procedures should be introduced or strengthened to prohibit sexual harassment, abuse and rape, including rape in marriage.

Laws which penalise homosexuality and prostitution should be repealed. The war on drugs should end, since it is a war on drug users and legitimises the alienation of users from the communities in which they live, inhibiting the effectiveness of health promotion and harm minimisation strategies. The criminal law affects the ability of drugs workers to provide adequate and appropriate health care, around sexual health and around the health implications of drug use itself.

Due attention needs to be paid to ensure that sexual health policies implemented in prisons and other closed institutions take full account of the principles set out in these recommendations.

Areas for international action and cooperation

Closer integration is needed between health promotion work in North Western and in Central and Eastern Europe.

Greater efforts are needed to bring together materials and approaches — videos, posters, evaluation reports etc — at supranational and national levels in accessible central stores, so that those entering the field later can learn from the mistakes and successes of earlier initiatives. Nevertheless, approaches must always be culturally specific and what works well in one context will not necessarily do so in another.

A condom research and information centre should be established which would coordinate information at WHO through the four programmes which have condoms on their agenda — the Global Programme on AIDS, the Maternal and Child Health programme, the Family Planning programme and the STDs programme — and interim findings from this condom centre should be published regularly in WHO newsletters.

A European standard for condoms is needed with a readily recognisable symbol which would appear on condom packets and on outlets through which condoms are available. There should be appropriate standards for condoms intended for vaginal and for anal intercourse, and manufacturers should diversify product ranges and undertake new marketing initiatives accordingly.

Urgent consultation is needed with Eastern European countries to develop appropriate responses to prevent sexual exploitation arising from economic imbalances between East and West.

Sexual health promotion strategy

Health promotion interventions need to be culturally specific, presenting sex in a positive light wherever possible, and in general designed and implemented with the active involvement of the intended target audience.

The objectives of HIV/AIDS prevention activities targetted at the general public are: firstly to sustain awareness, knowledge and risk reduction behaviour in the general population; and secondly, to create a social context which is favourable both to the care of those affected and the prevention of the further spread of the epidemic. This entails supporting and facilitating the work of those working with high risk behaviours, as well as legitimising the position of AIDS on the social and political agenda. *Hence, shift towards greater emphasis on more specified target audiences for HIV prevention should take place only hand in hand with continuation of broad spectrum approaches.*

Work with groups other than those directly targetted, eg parents, teachers, policy makers, and religious leaders, is important in order to create supportive environments for sexual health promotion. Opinion formers are, and should be, an essential component of all health programmes.

Health promotion should engage more forcefully with media, with politicians and with policy makers, not simply with target audiences themselves. Work to influence journalists and broadcast programme planners should be undertaken so that positive views of sexual health become more taken for granted in soap operas, current affairs programmes, etc.

Sex education should be organised both in formal and non-formal settings and *sex education in schools should be required by law.* Such education should aim at assisting the individual to develop the skills to benefit from freedom of choice and correctly assess risks to him/herself and others. It should include information about STDs and AIDS but not be restricted thereto.

Sustainability is an important consideration in mass media campaigns: in some countries this has been achieved through use of a constant theme — a logo, image, motif and slogan. Prevention workers should not assume that because they are bored with repetition of a message that a change of strategy is necessarily required.

Integration of HIV prevention, STD prevention and control, family planning and fertility control under the heading of sexual health is a good strategy in some respects, particularly in organisational terms, but is not without problems. These include: some practices promoted as "safer sex" for HIV prevention can transmit other STDs; problems of representing a coherent message to which people will want to listen.

Provision of voluntary testing, based upon informed consent and embedded in a range of services, should be upheld. Only in exceptional circumstances should the principle of medical confidentiality and the right not to know of HIV/STD infection be by-passed. Special provision should be made for minors, people with special needs, and those unable to express their own free will, to benefit from these principles.

Condoms need to be more widely available from a range of different outlets eg supermarkets, tobacconists, petrol stations and places where people meet. Practical skills in the correct use of condoms and lubricants need to be taught.

Gay communities should be recognised not as a target group for health promotion by agencies of the state, but an infrastructure for delivering health promotion effectively, both for gay men and for the larger group of men who have sex with men.

Primary health care is an important setting for sexual health promotion activities, and is particularly suited to integration of STD/HIV prevention with other aspects of sexual health, since primary health care providers are used to dealing with individuals in relationships and individuals in families rather than with separate conditions or diseases. Assessment of a client's health status should routinely include a sexual health dimension, recognising both the importance of human sexuality to individual health and the importance of a person's health status to their sexuality. Multi-disciplinary and inter-sectoral approaches should be developed within the framework of primary health care to deal more effectively with sexual health promotion.

Contraceptive providers should develop programmes within the framework of sexual health and appropriate to the communities they serve, which address issues such as the availability of social environments which support contraceptive use, independent decision making about unwanted pregnancy, STDs and HIV, and the abuse of power in sexual relationships.

Since sex and drugs issues cannot be wholly separated, integrated provision of needles, syringes and methadone with sexual health services is needed.

Recommendations for professional development and training

Coherent programmes are needed in initial teacher training and in-service education on sexual health education, and a national and local infrastructure should be created to support teachers involved in education for sexual health.

Training should be available for all staff working in reproductive health, sexual health and family planning services, which is relevant to their roles and emphasises their contribution to the work of a team. The goals of training should be to help workers become more aware of and comfortable with their own sexuality and the sexuality of others so that they are able to provide help in a non-judgmental manner.

Somatic, emotional, intellectual and social aspects of human sexuality should be components of basic professional training and education for primary health care providers. Continuing professional education in sexual health promotion should be developed based upon assessment of need and incorporated into existing frameworks where possible. Experience suggests that multi-disciplinary training and education is important in this context, as are allowing providers time out from their work to reflect and providing ongoing support through educators or facilitators who continue contact with providers to maintain their programmes of activity.

There are many issues which need to be addressed in terms of training of and support for drug workers to look at the full range of issues affecting drug users, including sexual health issues. Many such workers entered the field in the early 1980s as the "front line troops" in a war against drugs, and now need support in reorienting their work towards dealing with the complexities of problems of drug users, including their sexual health problems. Training and support to address sexual health issues should be an integral part of service strategy related to drug use. Training should provide a balance on theoretical, attitudinal and emotional issues and practical skills, whereas support must provide workers with the opportunity to address the emotional impact of the work in confidence, unlinked to supervision of performance and discipline.

Some health educators may require public relations training to enable them to become more effectively involved in political lobbying and media work.

One of the first principles of health promotion is providing a positive role model and all sexual health conferences and workshops should provide condoms to the delegates.

Recommendations relating to research needs and strategies for evaluating the success of health promotion initiatives

Evaluation of preventive activities should not simply be a sanctioning exercise, to demonstrate to politicians and funding bodies that particular initiatives have worked. It should also be possible to say that a project did not work, but that something was learnt from it.

Qualitative methods of evaluation are as important as quantitative, particularly in relation to change in the environment, ie the social and cultural context in which sexual health promotion takes place, which is not necessarily quantifiable. More eclectic methods of evaluation are needed in general, and especially new evaluative techniques for community initiatives.

The following research questions should be addressed by WHO and the European medical research councils: firstly to examine method and user failure and success rates of condoms in preventing unplanned pregnancy, transmission of HIV, and transmission of other STDs; secondly to investigate the user failure/success rates in behavioural and socio-economic context; thirdly, to examine and evaluate female barrier methods such as the female condom, spermicides, lubricants, condoms impregnated with spermicide, and dental dams.

Sound policy making and health promotion requires better quality information on the health status of minority ethnic people, collected and used with proper safeguards against abuse such as discrimination.

A code of conduct for researchers is urgently needed which reflects their societal responsibilities.

Recommendations relating to specific target audiences and contexts or settings for sexual health promotion

Women's power within the wider social and political context needs to be increased if lobbying and resetting of agendas is to be effective in terms of promoting women's sexual health.

There is an urgent need to target a group who tend to be overlooked when considering sexual health issues — men who have sex with women.

Governments should decriminalise homosexual behaviour and combat discrimination against lesbians and gay men, as a matter of both public health and human rights. In countries where gay communities are actually or almost non-existent, governments should encourage the creation of gay social venues. In schools, attention should be given to the problem of how to deal positively with gay and lesbian relationships and how to integrate such messages into the general context of sex and health education.

While some of the basic work now done by gay communities can be integrated into the mainstream, this will be neither cost-effective nor practically successful for all such initiatives.

The term "relapse" (into unsafe sexual behaviour) is unhelpful and potentially dangerous as a description of the complex factors underlying apparent increases in incidence of STDs among men who have sex with men. Gay communities and state agencies should initiate, develop and maintain cooperative research which identifies the real reasons behind the rise in STDs and should promulgate information on strategies to make sex both fulfilling and safe.

Drug users must be recognised as sexual beings representing the full range of human sexual experience, and should be afforded the same opportunities as the population as a whole to achieve sexual health.

Fear of stigmatisation must not be used as an excuse for inaction in relation to health promotion programmes and activities directed towards members of minority ethnic groups.

Sexual health promotion for ethnic minorities needs to be accurate, appropriate, culturally and linguistically sensitive with greater emphasis on oral and audiovisual technologies. Approaches include a more holistic view of health promotion not just focussing on STDs/HIV, and the involvement of minority ethnic groups in developing plans and programmes from an early stage. Collaboration between countries of origin and countries of residence may be helpful in developing health promotion strategies for some ethnic groups.

Education for young people needs to begin with their needs and the agendas they set. Young people should therefore determine the agenda for peer education, which should provide opportunities to talk with each other sensitively about sex and for self-reflection and re-examination of existing attitudes and beliefs.

There is room for developmental work in terms of supporting adolescent health care both within service provision and in the environment, since primary health care services have sometimes been poor in meeting the needs of adolescents. Creating a user-friendly environment includes removal of practical obstacles such as the cost and availability of services, condoms and other contraceptives.

It is essential that the sex industry is examined in a holistic context, which acknowledges the involvement of the numerous associated individuals and agencies, other than sex workers. All legal, social and political barriers to effective HIV prevention strategies within the sex industry need to be removed immediately.

Appendix 2: Committees and Contributors

International Advisory Committee

The Second International Workshop on Preventing the Sexual Transmission of HIV and other Sexually Transmitted Diseases was organised jointly by the UK Health Education Authority and the British Medical Association Foundation for AIDS. The organisers gratefully acknowledge the advice and assistance of the members of the International Advisory Committee, as follows:

Sir Donald Acheson	United Kingdom
Rafael de Andres Medina	Spain
Laura Ayres	Portugal
Nikolai Chaika	Union of Soviet Socialist Republics
Marianna Diomidis	Greece
Gauden Galea	Malta
Henning Jørgensen	Denmark
Lasse Kannas	Finland
Kurt Krikler	Austria
Bodil Langberg	Sweden
Peter Makara	Hungary
Hans Moerkerk	The Netherlands
Danielle Piette	Belgium
Hartmut Sasse	Italy
Zofia Słońska	Poland
Bertino Somaini	Switzerland
Kåre Tönnesen	Norway
James Walsh	Republic of Ireland

WHO Liason:

Svein-Erik Ekeid	Regional Office for Europe, Copenhagen
Rosmarie Erben	Headquarters, Geneva

EC Liaison:

Robin Gorna	Luxembourg

Organising Committee

Sîan Cosby	Health Education Authority, London
Hilary Curtis	British Medical Association Foundation for AIDS, London
Mukesh Kapila	Overseas Development Administration, London
Rosemary McMahon	Professional Briefings, London
Maria Paalman	Dutch Foundation for STD Control, Utrecht

Contributors

Professor Henriette Roscam Abbing: Vakgroep Gezondheidsrecht, Rijksuniversiteit Limburg, Postbus 616, 6200 MD Maastricht, The Netherlands.

Sir Donald Acheson KBE FRCP FRCS FFPHM FFOM: London School of Hygiene and Tropical Medicine, Keppel Street, London WC1E 7HT, United Kingdom.

Dr Peter Aggleton: Health and Education Research Unit, Goldsmith's College, Lewisham Way, New Cross, London SE14 6NW, United Kingdom.

Dr Peter Anderson: Primary Health Care Unit, Block 10, Churchill Hospital, Headington, Oxford OX3 7LJ, United Kingdom.

Renée Aroney: Kobler Center and John Hunter Clinic, Riverside Health Authority, 369 Fulham Road, London SW10 9HT, United Kingdom.

Virginia Blakey: Health Promotion Authority for Wales, Brunel House, 2 Fitzalan Road, Cardiff CF2 3LB, United Kingdom.

Dr Hilary Curtis: British Medical Association Foundation for AIDS, Tavistock Square, London WC1H 9JP, United Kingdom.

Peter Dankmeijer: Dutch Centre for Health Education and Health Promotion, Da Costakade 45, PO Box 5104, Utrecht 3502 JC, The Netherlands.

Dr William W Darrow PhD: Chief, Behavioral and Prevention Research Branch, Division of STD/HIV Prevention, National Center for Prevention Services, Centers for Disease Control, Public Health Service, US Department of Health and Human Services, Atlanta, Georgia 30333, USA.

Dr Peter Davies: Department of Sociology, University of Essex, Colchester CO4 3SQ, United Kingdom.

Michael Drummond: Centre for Health Economics, University of York, York YO1 5DD, United Kingdom.

Hugh Dufficy: SCODA (Standing Conference on Drug Abuse), 1-4 Hatton Place, London EC1N 8ND, United Kingdom.

Rinske van Duifhuizen MA: National Committee on AIDS Control, Polderweg 92, 1093 KP Amsterdam, The Netherlands.

Dr Svein-Erik Ekeid MB BS MA: WHO Regional Office for Europe, 8 Scherfigsvej, DK-2100 Copenhagen Ø, Denmark.

Dr Rosmarie Erben: WHO Regional Office for the Western Pacific, United Nations Avenue, PO Box 2932, Manila 2801, Philippines.

Christine Godfrey: Centre for Health Economics, University of York, York YO1 5DD, United Kingdom.

Marie Goldsmith: Health Education Authority, Hamilton House, Mabledon Place, London WC1H 9TX, United Kingdom.

Aart Hendriks LLM MA: Interfacultaire Werkgroep Homostudies, Rijksuniversiteir te Utrecht, Postbus 80140, 3508 TC Utrecht, The Netherlands.

Dr Margaret Jones: Brook Advisory Centres, 153a East Street, London SE17 2SD, United Kingdom.

Dr Tony Klouda: International Planned Parenthood Federation, PO Box 759, Inner Circle, Regent's Park, London NW1 4LQ, United Kingdom.

Dr Jan Kristoffersen MD: Skårer PHC Centre, Box 198, N-1473 Skårer, Norway.

Julian Meldrum: National AIDS Trust, Room 1403, Euston Tower, 286 Euston Road, London NW1 3DN, United Kingdom.

Ruth Morgan Thomas: Scot-PEP, 21a Torphichen Street, Edinburgh EH3 8HX, United Kingdom.

Maria Paalman: Dutch Foundation for STD Control, Catharijnesingel 56, 3511 GE Utrecht, The Netherlands.

Professor Peter Piot: WHO Collaborating Centre on AIDS, Institute of Tropical Medicine, Nationalestraat 155, 2000 Antwerpen, Belgium.

Professor Roger Short FRS: Department of Physiology, Monash University, Clayton, Melbourne, Victoria 3168, Australia.

Keith Tolley: Centre for Health Economics, University of York, York YO1 5DD, United Kingdom.

Dr Ronald O Valdiserri MD: Deputy Director (HIV), National Center for Prevention Services, Centers for Disease Control, Public Health Service, US Department of Health and Human Services, Atlanta, Georgia 30333, USA.

Kaye Wellings: Academic Department of Public Health, St Mary's Hospital Medical School, Praed Street, London W2 1PG, United Kingdom.